Abdominal Organ Transplantation

Abdominal Organ Transplantation

State of the Art

EDITED BY

Nizam Mamode

Consultant Transplant Surgeon
Reader in Transplant Surgery
Guy's and St Thomas' Hospital
Great Ormond Street Hospital
London, UK

Raja Kandaswamy

Professor and Vice-Chief
Division of Transplantation
Department of Surgery
University of Minnesota
Minneapolis, MN, USA

WILEY-BLACKWELL

A John Wiley & Sons, Ltd., Publication

Library of Congress Cataloging-in-Publication Data

Abdominal organ transplantation : state of the art / edited by Nizam Mamode,
Raja Kandaswamy.
    p. ; cm.
  Includes bibliographical references and index.
  ISBN 978-1-4443-3432-6 (cloth)
  I. Mamode, Nizam. II. Kandaswamy, Raja.
  [DNLM: 1. Abdomen–surgery. 2. Organ Transplantation–methods. WI 900]

  617.5′5059–dc23

                                                        2012026232

A catalogue record for this book is available from the British Library.

Wiley also publishes its books in a variety of electronic formats. Some content that appears in print may not be available in electronic books.

Cover design by : Nathan Harris

Set in 9.25/11.5pt Minion by Laserwords Private Limited, Chennai, India
Printed and bound in Malaysia by Vivar Printing Sdn Bhd

1 2013

Contents

List of Contributors

Adam D. Barlow
Specialist Registrar in General & Transplant Surgery
Department of Transplant Surgery
University Hospitals of Leicester
Leicester
UK

Anil Chandraker, MD, FASN, FRCP
Associate Professor of Medicine
Medical Director of Transplantation
Renal Division
Brigham and Women's Hospital
Harvard Medical School
Boston, MA
USA

Abhideep Chaudhary, MD, MBBS, MS
Clinical Fellow in Transplantation Surgery
University of Pittsburgh, Medical Center (UPMC)
Pittsburgh, PA
USA

Marc Clancy
Honorary Clinical Senior Lecturer
School of Medicine
University of Glasgow
Glasgow
UK

Chirag S. Desai, MD
Department of Surgery
University of Arizona College of Medicine
Tucson, AZ
USA

Steven Gabardi, PharmD, BCPS
Renal Division/Departments of Transplant Surgery and Pharmacy Services
Brigham and Women's Hospital and Department of Medicine
Harvard Medical School
Boston, MA
USA

Marc Gingell Littlejohn
Institute of Cancer Sciences
College of Medical, Veterinary and Life Sciences
University of Glasgow
Glasgow
UK

Rainer W.G. Gruessner, MD, FACS
Professor of Surgery and Immunology Chairman
Department of Surgery
University of Arizona College of Medicine
Tucson, AZ
USA

Abhinav Humar, MD
Professor of Surgery
University of Pittsburgh, Medical Center (UPMC)
Pittsburgh, PA
USA

Tun Jie, MD, MS, FACS
Assistant Professor of Surgery
General Surgery/Abdominal Transplant/Hepatopancreatic and biliary
  Surgery
Department of Surgery
University of Arizona College of Medicine
Tucson, AZ
USA

**Paul R.V. Johnson, MBChB, MA, MD, FRCS(Eng +Edin),
  FRCS(Paed.Surg), FAAP**
Professor of Paediatric Surgery University of Oxford
Director of DRWF Human Islet Isolation Facility and Oxford Islet
  Transplant Programme
Consultant Paediatric Surgeon
John Radcliffe Hospital
Fellow at St Edmund Hall
University of Oxford
Oxford
UK

Maciej T. Juszczak
Islet Transplant Programme, Oxford Centre for Diabetes, Endocrinology
    and Metabolism, and Islet Transplant Research Group
Nuffield Department of Surgical Sciences
University of Oxford
Oxford
UK

Raja Kandaswamy, MD, FACS
Professor and Vice-Chief, Division of Transplantation
Department of Surgery
University of Minnesota
Minneapolis, MN
USA

Khalid M. Khan, MBChB, MRCP
Associate Professor Director
Pediatric Liver & Intestine Transplant Program
University of Arizona
Tucson, AZ
USA

Nizam Mamode, BSc, MB ChB, MD, FRCS, FRCS(Gen)
Consultant Transplant Surgeon
Reader in Transplant Surgery
Guy's and St Thomas' Hospital
Great Ormond Street Hospital
London
UK

Stephen D. Marks, MD, MSc, MRCP, DCH, FRCPCH
Consultant Paediatric Nephrologist
Department of Paediatric Nephrology
Great Ormond Street Hospital for Children NHS Trust
London
UK

Michael L. Nicholson, MD, DSc, FRCS
Professor of Transplant Surgery
Department of Transplant Surgery
University Hospitals of Leicester
Leicester
UK

Leonardo V. Riella, MD, PhD
Instructor in Medicine
Transplant Research Center
Renal Division
Brigham and Women's Hospital
Harvard Medical School
Boston, MA
USA

Paul G. Shiels
Department of Surgery
University of Glasgow
Western Infirmary Glasgow
Glasgow
UK

Rajinder Singh
Consultant Transplant Surgeon
Guy's and St Thomas' Hospital
Great Ormond Street Hospital
London
UK

Karen S. Stevenson
Institute of Cancer Sciences
College of Medical, Veterinary and Life Sciences
University of Glasgow
Glasgow
UK

David E.R. Sutherland, MD, PhD
Professor
Department of Surgery
University of Minnesota
Minneapolis, MN
USA

Foreword

This miscellaneous collection of articles on new developments in organ transplantation will be of very considerable interest to organ transplant clinicians. The chapters range from living donation of the kidney and liver to intestinal and pancreas the kidney, with a very good chapter on new surgical techniques in transplantation. In addition there is a comprehensive chapter on ABO incompatible renal transplantation and transplantation in the patient that is highly sensitized to HLA. There is a short review of the current status of pancreatic islet transplantation as well as an extensive review of new developments in pancreas transplantation. Furthermore paediatric renal transplantation is well covered and there are interesting contributions on novel cell therapies in transplantation as well as on immunosuppressive therapies, concentrating on more recent developments in this area. The final chapter by the two editors reviews the status of renal, liver, pancreas and intestinal transplantation, but in particular outlines the problems that still have to be resolved. The editors recognise that the current one year graft survival rates are at a level that was not considered remotely possible even as little as 20 years ago but accept that the longer term outcomes are still disappointing despite the introduction of many new immunosuppressive strategies. But in general they are very optimistic about the future.

Overall this book will be considered a very good read by the transplant clinician.

Sir Peter J Morris AC, FRS
Director, Centre for Evidence in Transplantation,
Royal College of Surgeons of England and London School of Hygiene and Tropical Medicine.
Emeritus Nuffield Professor of Surgery, University of Oxford.
Past President, Royal college of Surgeons.
Honorary Professor, University of London.

1 Living Donation: The Gold Standard

Leonardo V. Riella and Anil Chandraker
Renal Division, Brigham and Women's Hospital, Harvard Medical School, USA

Introduction

The first successful transplant occurred in Boston in 1954, when a surgical team under the direction of Joseph Murray removed a kidney from a healthy donor and transplanted it into his identical twin, who had chronic glomerulonephritis [1]. The organ functioned immediately and the recipient survived for 9 years, after which time his allograft failed from what was thought to be recurrent glomerulonephritis. More than 50 years have passed since that breakthrough achievement, and transplantation has progressed from an experimental modality to standard of care. The introduction of immunosuppressive drugs such as azathioprine, prednisone, and later calcineurin inhibitors has led to better outcomes and, along with technical breakthroughs, expanded the pool of organs available to deceased and human leukocyte antigen (HLA)-mismatched donors.

Kidney transplantation has become the preferred therapeutic option for patients with end-stage kidney disease (ESKD), leading to better patient survival and quality of life. It is also more cost-effective than dialysis [2–4]. Unfortunately, the incidence of ESKD has risen steadily in the past several decades, creating a shortage of available organs for patients on the kidney-transplant waiting list (Table 1.1).

This growth in ESKD is related to the increased incidence of diabetes, obesity, and hypertension, combined with the improvement in treatment for concurrent health problems such as ischemic heart disease and stroke. The supply of organs from deceased donors has not followed the same upward trend, resulting in an ever-widening gap between eligible potential transplant recipients and available organs (Table 1.2).

In 2009, only 18% of patients on the waiting list for kidney transplantation received an organ [5]. The average waiting time for kidneys from deceased donors in the USA is more than 3 years, and in some geographic areas it is more than 5 years (Table 1.3)—waiting times that are sometimes longer than the average life expectancy of middle-aged and older persons with ESKD [6]. In line with these numbers, a recent study indicates that even

Abdominal Organ Transplantation: State of the Art, First Edition.
Edited by Nizam Mamode and Raja Kandaswamy.
© 2013 Blackwell Publishing Ltd. Published 2013 by Blackwell Publishing Ltd.

Table 1.1 Waiting list for different organs in the USA. OPTN, Organ Procurement and Transplantation Network. Data from [5].

Waiting list candidates OPTN 2010	Number
All	107,075
Kidney	84,495
Pancreas	1,458
Kidney/Pancreas	2,182
Liver	15,948
Intestine	248
Heart	3,173
Lung	1,844
Heart/Lung	75

Table 1.2 Growth of the kidney-transplant waiting list compared to donor type in the USA. Data from [5].

	2009	1999	1989
Waiting List	84,495	40,825	17,786
All type donors	14,631	10,862	5,929
Deceased Donors	8,021	5,824	4,011
Living Donors	6,610	5,038	1,918
% Living donors	45%	46%	32%

Table 1.3 Time to transplant by organ type in the USA. Data from [5].

Organ type	Time to transplant in 2004 (median in days)
Kidney	1,219
Pancreas Transplant Alone	376
Pancreas after Kidney	562
Kidney-Pancreas	149
Liver	400
Intestine	212
Heart	166
Lung	792

major alterations in the organ procurement process cannot reasonably be expected to meet the demand for transplantable kidneys from decreased donors [7]. The imbalance between patient demand and the supply of organs from deceased donors has refocused attention on living kidney donors.

Epidemiology

Living-donor kidney transplantation is rapidly increasing in popularity worldwide and has surpassed the number of deceased donors in many transplant centers [5]. In 2009, approximately 40% of all kidney donations were from living donors, and most major transplant centers in the USA have been increasing the proportion of living donors, reaching more than 60% of total transplants in some. However, wide variations exist worldwide in the use of living and deceased kidney donors. These differences reflect varying medical, ethical, social, and cultural values, as well as the availability of deceased-donor organs. For example, Spain has possibly the most efficient system of deceased-organ collection, with less than 5% of transplants being from living donors. At the other end of the spectrum, strong cultural barriers in Japan have led to a preponderance of living-organ transplantation. Similarly, Turkey and Greece rely mainly on living donation as a source of organ transplantation [8].

Several factors have influenced the expansion of living donation. The advent of laparoscopic nephrectomy has reduced the associated morbidity of kidney removal, making more donors receptive to an interruption of the healthy course of their lives. Just as importantly, epidemiological data have shown that irrespective of the HLA match or the donor–recipient relationship, recipients of living-donor kidneys (LDKs) fare better than those who receive deceased-donor kidneys (DDKs) (Figure 1.1). Finally, the development of stronger immunosuppression and desensitization techniques has overcome many of the biological barriers to successful transplantation,

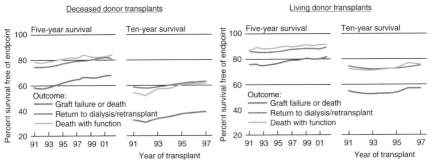

Figure 1.1 Outcomes of kidney transplants according to donor type. Graft-survival estimates are adjusted for age, gender, race, and primary diagnosis, using Cox proportional-hazards models. Conditional half-life estimates depend on first-year graft survival. (Reproduced from [6] The data reported here have been supplied by the United States Renal Data System (USRDS). The interpretation and reporting of these data are the responsibility of the author(s) and in no way should be seen as an official policy or interpretation of the U.S. government)

such as ABO incompatibility or the presence of low to medium titers of antidonor HLA antibodies (Abs). Today, any person who is well and willing to donate may potentially be a live-kidney donor.

Advantages of living-kidney donation

It is well recognized that renal dysfunction is associated with accelerated heart disease. It has been estimated that mortality associated with cardiovascular disease is increased approximately 10-fold among patients with ESKD, even after accounting for age, sex, race, and the presence of diabetes [9]. Successful kidney transplantation progressively reduces the incidence of cardiac mortality and is therefore associated with an overall survival benefit in subjects undergoing kidney transplantation [10]. Even in older transplant recipients and patients with ESKD secondary to diabetes or obesity—subgroups with higher perioperative cardiovascular complications—survival benefits persist [4,11].

One-year survival for a functioning transplant is 90% for recipients of deceased-donor transplants and 96% for recipients of transplants from living donors. After surviving the first year with a functioning transplant, 50% of recipients of deceased- and living-donor transplants are projected to be alive with a functioning transplant at 13 and 23 years, respectively.

The waiting time on dialysis has emerged as one of the strongest independent modifiable risk factors for poor renal-transplant outcome [12], as can be seen in Figure 1.2. The presumed negative effect of prolonged dialysis is likely related to the impact of ESKD on cardiovascular morbidity and is observed in both living- and deceased-kidney recipients. However, even after a prolonged wait, patients who eventually receive a kidney transplant still have a lower mortality than those who continued on dialysis [13]. The possibility of undergoing preemptive transplantation without the need for dialysis gives the ESKD patients the best possible outcome [13–15]. With these observations in mind, until an optimal and timely source of organs is developed to decrease the prolonged waiting times, living-kidney-donor transplantation provides the best alternative for most patients [13–15].

Living-kidney donation is an act of profound human generosity and can be a source of much gratification for all parties involved. Many donors describe it as the most meaningful experience of their lives and the quality of life of donors after transplantation is reported to be better than or equivalent to that of controls [16]. Nonetheless, given the highly asymmetric nature of the physical benefits arising from kidney donation, a careful psychiatric evaluation of the donor is essential, to assess the coercion-free, informed, and autonomous decision to proceed with the process.

The number of sensitized recipients has increased dramatically in the past couple of years and these recipients usually face the greatest waiting times, due to the presence of preformed antibodies, and consequently have the greatest mortality. Desensitization protocols have enabled them to plan and receive an LDK at a determined time, but these protocols are expensive

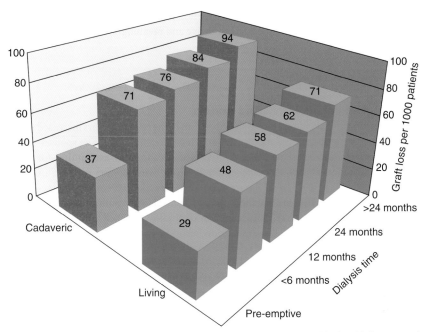

Figure 1.2 Comparison of rates of graft loss associated with living- and deceased (cadaveric)-donor transplantation according to time on dialysis prior to transplantation [12]. (Reproduced from [12], Copyright © 2002, (C) 2002 Lippincott Williams)

and labor-intensive, and in the USA have been implemented only for small numbers of patients. While successful in the short-term, the long-term outcomes remain unknown; these techniques are discussed further in Chapter 5. Another potential option for such patients is a paired-kidney exchange (PKE), which is discussed in more detail later in this chapter. For many years, immunological barriers were thought to be the largest hurdle in transplantation; today, many cite the acute shortage of organs as the major limitation.

Finally, the administration of donor-derived cells into the recipient in order to induce immunological hyporesponsiveness to the solid-organ transplant and minimize the need for immunosuppression has recently been explored. This hyporesponsiveness was thought to occur due to the generation of mixed chimerism, immune deviation, and/or generation of a regulatory immunological phenotype. Kawai *et al.* have recently published a report on a small number of successful cases of combined bone-marrow and kidney transplant in HLA single-haplotype mismatched, living, related donors, with the use of a nonmyeloablative preparative regimen. Four out of five recipients were able to discontinue all immunosuppressive therapy 14 months after transplantation, opening new possibilities for the induction of transplant tolerance with living-kidney donation, with consequent improvement in long-term outcomes [17].

In summary, living donation provides one answer to the shortage of donor organs, allows preemptive transplantation, and leads to better long-term graft survival. It also permits the introduction of new, tolerogenic strategies, and for many donors will be a very positive and meaningful experience.

Types of donor

Related versus unrelated donors

Whereas rates of kidney transplantation from living related donors increased during the 1990s, transplantation from living unrelated (including spousal) donors has increased rapidly over the past decade, now accounting for nearly one-quarter of all transplantations from living donors in the USA (Figure 1.3). In 1995, a landmark report by Terasaki and colleagues documented that HLA-mismatched spousal transplants resulted in a graft survival superior to that of anything but identically matched kidneys from deceased donors [14]. This observation has influenced decisions regarding the suitability of live donors who are spouses, friends of the recipient, or anonymous; there is little concern today about the degree of HLA matching for the crossmatch-negative recipient of a kidney from a living donor. With directed donation to loved ones or friends, concerns have arisen about the intense pressure that can be put on people to donate, leading those who are reluctant to do so to feel coerced. Donor evaluation by a team of physicians other than that treating the recipient and a focus on the donor's interests when evaluating for donation minimize these risks. Furthermore, the general approach of simply reporting an unwilling donor as 'unsuitable' is a safe method of protecting the donor's decision without harming their relationship with the recipient.

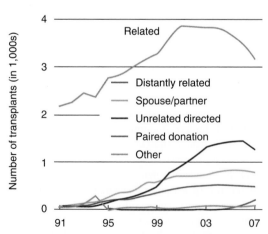

Figure 1.3 Number of transplants from living donors, by donor relation. (Reproduced from [6] The data reported here have been supplied by the United States Renal Data System (USRDS). The interpretation and reporting of these data are the responsibility of the author(s) and in no way should be seen as an official policy or interpretation of the U.S. government)

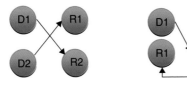

Two Pair Exchange   Three Pair Exchange

Figure 1.4 Examples of paired-kidney exchange (PKE). The traditional two-pair exchange is shown on the left, while a more complex three-pair exchange is shown on the right. The latter occurs when one of the donors is incompatible with the reciprocal matched recipient. The three pairs can be arranged so that donor kidneys are simultaneously exchanged from pairs 1 to 2, 2 to 3, and 3 to 1. D, donor; R, recipient

Paired-kidney exchange

When available donors are incompatible with their intended recipients due to ABO or HLA antibodies, many transplant centers participate in kidney live-donor paired-exchange programs [18–20]. In a conventional PKE donation (two-way exchange), two donor–recipient pairs surmount each other's incompatibility problem by simply exchanging donors (Figure 1.4). To ensure that both recipients receive their grafts, the two transplantations are arranged simultaneously. The probability of finding a suitable donor–recipient pair for an exchange is greatly influenced by the pool size. Even in a successful large national PKE program, only around 50% of incompatible pairs usually find a match and undergo a transplant—primarily due to the blood-group imbalance in the pool of incompatible pairs [21]. There is a predominance of group A donors and group O recipients. National matching programs would make the likelihood of finding pairs greater and would likely expand this type of organ transplantation.

PKEs have been performed in the USA for nearly a decade, as either single-center or, increasingly, multiregional programs. A recent report showed that only 334 paired donations had been carried out in the USA since 2000 [22]. Legal and logistical barriers have been regarded as some of the major reasons for this poor success. Mutiregional data-sharing has substantially impacted PKE transplants [23]. There are now a number of regional PKE programs within the United Network for Organ Sharing (UNOS), such as the New England Program for Kidney Exchange (NEPKE), with 14 transplant centers in region 2, and the Alliance for Paired Donation, a 22-state coalition of 65 transplant programs. We believe a centralized national PKE program would give the greatest potential for matching incompatible donors. Such national schemes are currently operating in the Netherlands and the UK. The Dutch have reported numerous challenges and barriers in their exchange program, and a flexible organization was key to creating alternative solutions [20]. The rate of kidney transplantation can be increased by an average of 7–15% with a PKE program [24]. A recent study by the Dutch program suggested that the optimal chain length for living-kidney donation is three [25]. In the UK experience, the use of altruistic, nondirected donors to start a chain of transplants may offer the greatest potential to increase the number of successful paired-kidney-donation transplants [26].

Altruistic donors

The success of living unrelated kidney transplantation has influenced transplant physicians to sanction the requests of individuals who wish to be anonymous donors; that is, "nondirected or altruistic donors" [27]. The motives of the nondirected donor should be established with care in order to avoid a prospective donor's intention of remedying a psychological disorder via donation. In general, these kidneys are allocated according to the waiting list for deceased-kidney donors [27]. Some centers advocate the allocation of such organs into a PKE program, since this can result in a domino effect and facilitate multiple transplants [23,28]. Directed donation to a stranger—whereby donors choose to give to a specific person with whom they have no prior emotional connection—is generally not supported, primarily because of fears of commercial incentive or psychological coercion [29].

Organ commercialism, which targets vulnerable populations (such as illiterate and impoverished persons, undocumented immigrants, prisoners, and political or economic refugees) in resource-poor countries, has been condemned by international bodies such as the World Health Organization (WHO) for decades. In recent years, as a consequence of the increasing ease of Internet communication and the willingness of patients in rich countries to travel to purchase organs, organ trafficking and transplant tourism have grown into global problems. For example, as of 2006, foreigners received two-thirds of the 2000 kidney transplants performed annually in Pakistan [30].

An international transplantation summit was held in Istanbul in 2008, which resulted in the "Declaration of Istanbul on Organ Trafficking and Transplant Tourism" [30–33]. This proclaims that the poor who sell their organs are being exploited, whether by richer people within their own country or by transplant tourists from abroad. Moreover, transplant tourists risk physical harm by unregulated and illegal transplantation. Participants in the Istanbul summit concluded that transplant commercialism, transplant tourism, and organ trafficking should be prohibited. They also urged their fellow transplant professionals, individually and through their organizations, to put an end to these unethical activities and foster safe, accountable practices that meet the needs of transplant recipients while protecting donors.

Evaluation process for the live donor

Living donation appears contrary to the most fundamental concept of the medical profession: *"primum non nocere"* ("first, do no harm"). It exposes a healthy individual to the combined risks of major surgery and life with a single kidney entirely for the benefit of another person. With that in mind,

LDK transplantation should only be undertaken if five essential conditions are met:

- The risk to the donor is low.
- The donor is fully informed of the risks and benefits as a donor
- The donor is medically and psychosocially suitable.
- The decision to donate is voluntary and entirely without coercion.
- The transplant has a good chance of providing a successful outcome for the recipient.

The Amsterdam consensus statement emphasizes that the purpose of the evaluation process is to ensure the overall health and well-being of the donor, minimizing unnecessary medical risk to both donor and recipient [34]. It should quantify any potential technical difficulties that might compromise the success of the nephrectomy and subsequent transplantation.

By general consensus, the optimal donor is an adult member of the immediate family of a patient with ESKD [29]. However, the use of emotionally related but genetically unrelated living donors has become increasingly common worldwide, and this practice is supported by different guidelines.

It is generally accepted that children (under the age of 18) should not donate. As can be seen in Table 1.4, the majority of donors in the USA are between 35 and 49 years old; nonetheless, the upper age limit has been advancing in recent years. There are no set guidelines for an upper age limit for donation, but most centers accept donors up to 70 years of age, after a thorough investigation for underlying kidney disease, latent cardiovascular disease, or malignancy.

A written informed consent is mandatory in most countries, with the understanding that consent can be withdrawn at any time. Moreover, the donor evaluation should ideally be undertaken by a physician who is not directly involved with the proposed transplantation or the recipient's care, in order to avoid any bias in the process. If the potential donor decides not to donate, the recipient is usually told that the donor is 'unsuitable'; detailed information should not be given, nor should untrue statements be

Table 1.4 Number of kidney donors by age in the USA. Data from [5].

	2009	2008	2007	2006	2005
All Ages	6,388	5,968	6,043	6,435	6,571
6–10 Years	0	0	0	0	0
11–17 Years	3	0	0	1	0
18–34 Years	1,937	1,849	1,872	2,034	2,078
35–49 Years	2,746	2,593	2,675	2,938	3,103
50–64 Years	1,595	1,437	1,415	1,390	1,332
65 +	107	89	81	71	58

made. Some controversial positions might arise when recipients are HIV positive and the potential live-related donor is not aware of the recipient's HIV status. The UK guidelines specify that the donor has the right to know the HIV status of the recipient in order to have a fully informed consent [35]. Others might argue that it is essential to inform the donor about the high-risk status of the recipient, but it is not necessary to give additional medical details about the recipient's condition.

The financial aspects of donation should be discussed, due to the important implications early after transplant. The future donor must be aware of any expenses involved with the surgery and postsurgical care, as well as the loss of income in the first few weeks after transplant, where activity is limited. The latter is minimized significantly by the use of a laparoscopic approach to harvesting the donor kidney. Moreover, congressional legislation in the USA has provided an important model to remove financial disincentives to being a live donor: federal employees are now afforded paid leave and coverage for travel expenses.

During the initial evaluation, the potential donor is assessed for any obvious medical or psychosocial contraindication to donation in order to avoid unnecessary further investigation. Some laboratory information is also collected during this first visit, including serum creatinine, blood count, urine dipstick, and ABO/HLA typing. The major contraindications for kidney donation are known diabetes, significant hypertension or proteinuria, a glomerular filtration rate (GFR) below the stated acceptable value for age, active infection, active malignancy, and recurrent kidney stones [36]. Serology for infectious diseases, chest x-ray (CXR), electrocardiogram (ECG), purified protein derivative (PPD) skin test for tuberculosis, and cancer screening exams appropriate for age are also performed. As a final step, renal imaging is done, typically with a computed tomography (CT) angiogram, in order to assess kidney size, the renal vessels, and the urinary tract. More details of the donor evaluation process can be found in [34] and [36].

Obesity in not considered a contraindication in either US or European guidelines, but it has been documented that a body mass index (BMI) over 30 significantly increases the perioperative complication rate, and some concerns exist about the long-term consequences of nephrectomy.

The evaluation for hypertension should include blood pressure (BP) measurements by an experienced provider on three separate occasions; verification of elevated levels should be undertaken with ambulatory BP monitoring as approximately 10–20% may be found to have normal BP [37,38]. If elevated BP is detected and the prospective donor is still under consideration, a CXR, ECG, echocardiogram, and ophthalmologic evaluation should be performed to look for secondary consequences of hypertension. In addition, a 24-hour urine collection for albumin excretion or a spot urine for albumin–creatinine ratio should be performed, along with a urinalysis and a formal GFR measurement. If donors with hypertension donate, they should be followed longitudinally by the transplant center to ensure optimal treatment and monitoring of complications. Overall, hypertensive donors are increasingly being used in transplant centers due to the limited availability of organs; however, more detailed information about these donors and their long-term outcomes is needed before they can be generally accepted [38,39].

GFR tends to decrease with age, with an approximately 10 ml/minute drop per decade after age 40. In general, it seems prudent to require living donors to have a GFR at the average of the age-specific GFR [40]. In obese and elderly patients, GFR cannot be estimated accurately with the Cockroft–Gault or Modification of Diet in Renal Disease (MDRD) equations [40]. The majority of centers use a radioisotope exam to estimate the GFR (e.g. $^{51}Cr\ EDTA$) and assess this against the lower limit for the age of the donor, which can be seen in Table 1.5 and Figure 1.5 [36,41].

Table 1.5 Acceptable glomerular filtration rate (GFR) by donor age prior to donation. Data from [5].

Donor age (years)	Acceptable corrected GFR prior to donation (ml/min/1.73 m²)
Up to 46	80
50	77
60	68
70	59
80	50

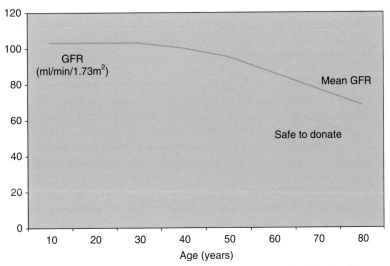

Figure 1.5 Graph of acceptable GFR by donor age prior to donation [36]. (Reproduced from http://www.renal.org /Libraries/Other_Guidlines/BTS_and_RA_Guideline_on_Living_Donor_Kidney_Transplantation_3rd_Edition_April _2011.sflb.ashx with permission from The British Transplantation Society and The Renal Association)

Short-term and long-term risks of kidney donation

The donor must be fully informed of the risks of surgery: donor nephrectomy is associated with a very low perioperative risk, with mortality of 0.03% being commonly reported [42]. It has been suggested that the risk can be compared with that of dying in a car accident during the next year, to enable potential donors to grasp the practical meaning of such an incidence rate. Laparoscopic nephrectomy now accounts for >50% of the donor nephrectomy procedures in the USA [43]. This technique has led to shorter hospital stays (2–4 days, compared with 3–7), less incisional discomfort, and an earlier return to work (12–21 days, compared with 30–60) than after open procedures [43–45]. Bleeding was the most common reason for reoperation after non-hand-assisted laparoscopic donation [45]. The most important perioperative risks due to donor nephrectomy include atelectasis, pneumothorax, pneumonia, urinary-tract infection (UTI), wound complications, and deep vein thrombosis with or without pulmonary embolism. In a cohort of 2509 living-donor nephrectomies, the risk of major morbidity for all donors was 4.9% (laparoscopic = 4.5%, open = 5.1%, p = 0.549) and the overall rate of any morbidity was 14.3% (laparoscopic = 10.3%, open = 15.7%, p = 0.001) [46].

The first study to attest the long-term safety of unilateral nephrectomy came from sixty-two World War II veterans who had undergone nephrectomy owing to trauma [47]. Mortality was not increased and autopsy results available in 20 cases did not show any evidence of glomerulosclerosis. More recent studies have confirmed no significant risk to the kidney donors up to 35 years after nephrectomy [42,48]. Decline in renal function parallels that of age-related healthy individuals with two kidneys. Urine albumin excretion, attributable to single-nephron hyperfiltration from reduced renal mass, may be elevated but is usually low-grade and not associated with higher risk for renal dysfunction.

The largest trial included 3698 kidney donors with a mean of 12 years of follow-up [48]. The population studied was very healthy, with no evidence of hypertension or proteinuria (<200 mg/day). There was no difference in the incidence of ESKD, hypertension, or renal dysfunction when compared to controls matched for age, sex, and race. There was also no survival difference when compared to controls from the general population. However, the time since donation was significantly associated with the development of albuminuria. The subgroup that was compared to controls represented mainly Caucasians (99%), with a predominance of females (60%). Extrapolation of the results to African Americans, Latinos, and South Asians, subgroups in whom chronic kidney disease tends to progress more rapidly, is not reasonable. One of the issues with using the general population as the comparative group is that kidney donors are a preselected group of patients with no significant medical comorbidities and excellent survival to start with, leading to a selection bias and possibly masking a potential deleterious effect of organ donation.

Nonetheless, the published evidence indicates that there is little long-term medical risk to a healthy donor after unilateral nephrectomy. However, the profile of the donor has recently changed to include those with isolated medical abnormalities such as hypertension, an increased BMI, dyslipidemia, and stone disease [19]. Further validation is necessary to ensure these donors do not see significant consequences from having a single kidney later in life.

Conclusion

Living-kidney-donor transplantation provides the best alternative for most patients with advanced chronic kidney disease. Due to the shortage of deceased kidney donors and the increased prevalence of ESKD, rates of living donation will continue to increase in the near future. In addition, innovative approaches that allow incompatible donor recipients to undergo transplantation are being developed, increasing the pool of potential organ recipients. Nonetheless, donor safety should always be kept in mind and we strongly advocate for the creation of national donor registries, which will allow close monitoring of the donors in the long term and ensure the preservation of our fundamental rule of "*primum non nocere.*"

References

1 Merrill JP, Murray JE, Harrison JH, Guild WR. Successful homotransplantation of the human kidney between identical twins. *J Am Med Assoc* 1956;160(4):277–282.

2 Laupacis A, Keown P, Pus N, Krueger H, Ferguson B, Wong C, *et al.* A study of the quality of life and cost-utility of renal transplantation. *Kidney Int* 1996;50(1):235–242.

3 Evans RW, Manninen DL, Garrison LP Jr,, Hart LG, Blagg CR, Gutman RA, *et al.* The quality of life of patients with end-stage renal disease. *N Engl J Med* 1985;312(9):553–559.

4 Wolfe RA, Ashby VB, Milford EL, Ojo AO, Ettenger RE, Agodoa LY, *et al.* Comparison of mortality in all patients on dialysis, patients on dialysis awaiting transplantation, and recipients of a first cadaveric transplant. *N Engl J Med* 1999;341(23):1725–1730.

5 OPTN Organ Procurement and Transplantation Network Database. http://optn.transplant.hrsa.gov/data/ [accessed 04/01/2010]. 2010; US Department of Health and Human Services.

6 US Renal Data System. USRDS 2009 Annual Data Report: Atlas of End-Stage Renal Disease in the United States. http://www.usrds.org/2009/pres/SA_FC346_mortality_10_31_09.pdf [accessed 04/15/2010]. 2009; Bethesda, MD: National Institutes of Health, National Institute of Diabetes and Digestive and Kidney Diseases.

7 Sheehy E, Conrad SL, Brigham LE, Luskin R, Weber P, Eakin M, *et al.* Estimating the number of potential organ donors in the United States. *N Engl J Med* 2003;349(7):667–674.

8 Price D. Living kidney donation in Europe: legal and ethical perspectives—the EUROTOLD Project. *Transplant International* 2008;7(S1):665–667.

9 Sarnak MJ, Levey AS. Cardiovascular disease and chronic renal disease: a new paradigm. *Am J Kidney Dis* 2000;35(4 Suppl 1):S117–S131.

10 Meier-Kriesche HU, Schold JD, Srinivas TR, Reed A, Kaplan B. Kidney transplantation halts cardiovascular disease progression in patients with end-stage renal disease. *Am J Transplant* 2004;4(10):1662–1668.

11 Glanton CW, Kao TC, Cruess D, Agodoa LY, Abbott KC. Impact of renal transplantation on survival in end-stage renal disease patients with elevated body mass index. *Kidney Int* 2003;63(2):647–653.

12 Meier-Kriesche HU, Kaplan B. Waiting time on dialysis as the strongest modifiable risk factor for renal transplant outcomes: a paired donor kidney analysis. *Transplantation* 2002;74(10):1377–1381.

13 Meier-Kriesche HU, Port FK, Ojo AO, Rudich SM, Hanson JA, Cibrik DM, *et al*. Effect of waiting time on renal transplant outcome. *Kidney Int* 2000;58(3):1311–1317.

14 Terasaki PI, Cecka JM, Gjertson DW, Takemoto S. High survival rates of kidney transplants from spousal and living unrelated donors. *N Engl J Med* 1995;333(6):333–336.

15 Mange KC, Joffe MM, Feldman HI. Effect of the use or nonuse of long-term dialysis on the subsequent survival of renal transplants from living donors. *N Engl J Med* 2001;344(10):726–731.

16 Fehrman-Ekholm I, Brink B, Ericsson C, Elinder CG, Duner F, Lundgren G. Kidney donors don't regret: follow-up of 370 donors in Stockholm since 1964. *Transplantation* 2000;69(10):2067–2071.

17 Kawai T, Cosimi AB, Spitzer TR, Tolkoff-Rubin N, Suthanthiran M, Saidman SL, *et al*. HLA-mismatched renal transplantation without maintenance immunosuppression. *N Engl J Med*. 2008;358(4):353–361.

18 Montgomery RA, Zachary AA, Ratner LE, Segev DL, Hiller JM, Houp J, *et al*. Clinical results from transplanting incompatible live kidney donor/recipient pairs using kidney paired donation. *JAMA* 2005;294(13):1655–1663.

19 Davis CL, Delmonico FL. Living-donor kidney transplantation: a review of the current practices for the live donor. *J Am Soc Nephrol* 2005;16(7):2098–2110.

20 de Klerk M, Keizer KM, Claas FH, Witvliet M, Haase-Kromwijk BJ, Weimar W. The Dutch national living donor kidney exchange program. *Am J Transplant* 2005;5(9):2302–2305.

21 de Klerk M, Witvliet MD, Haase-Kromwijk BJ, Claas FH, Weimar W. A highly efficient living donor kidney exchange program for both blood type and crossmatch incompatible donor-recipient combinations. *Transplantation* 2006;82(12):1616–1620.

22 Hanto RL, Reitsma W, Delmonico FL. The development of a successful multiregional kidney paired donation program. *Transplantation* 2008;86(12):1744–1748.

23 Ferrari P, de Klerk M. Paired kidney donations to expand the living donor pool. *J Nephrol* 2009;22(6):699–707.

24 de Klerk M, Weimar W. Ingredients for a successful living donor kidney exchange program. *Transplantation* 2008;86(4):511–512.

25 De Klerk M, Van Der Deijl WM, Witvliet MD, Haase-Kromwijk BJ, Claas FH, Weimar W. The optimal chain length for kidney paired exchanges: an analysis of the Dutch program. *Transpl Int* 2010;23(11):1120–1125.

26 Johnson RJ, Allen JE, Fuggle SV, Bradley JA, Rudge C. Early experience of paired living kidney donation in the United kingdom. *Transplantation* 2008;86(12):1672–1677.

27 Matas AJ, Garvey CA, Jacobs CL, Kahn JP. Nondirected donation of kidneys from living donors. *N Engl J Med* 2000;343(6):433–436.

28 Rees MA, Kopke JE, Pelletier RP, Segev DL, Rutter ME, Fabrega AJ, *et al.* A nonsimultaneous, extended, altruistic-donor chain. *N Engl J Med* 2009; 360(11):1096–1101.

29 Kasiske BL, Ravenscraft M, Ramos EL, Gaston RS, Bia MJ, Danovitch GM; Ad Hoc Clinical Practice Guidelines Subcommittee of the Patient Care and Education Committee of the American Society of Transplant Physicians. *The evaluation of living renal transplant donors: clinical practice guidelines. J Am Soc Nephrol* 1996;7(11):2288–2313.

30 The Declaration of Istanbul on Organ Trafficking and Transplant Tourism. *Clin J Am Soc Nephrol* 2008;3(5):1227–1231.

31 Reed AI, Merion RM, Roberts JP, Klintmalm GB, Abecassis MM, Olthoff KM, *et al.* The Declaration of Istanbul: review and commentary by the American Society of Transplant Surgeons Ethics Committee and Executive Committee. *Am J Transplant* 2009;9(11):2466–2469.

32 The Declaration of Istanbul on organ trafficking and transplant tourism. *Kidney Int* 2008;74(7):854–859.

33 The Declaration of Istanbul on Organ Trafficking and Transplant Tourism. Istanbul Summit April 30–May 2, 2008. Nephrol Dial Transplant 2008;23(11): 3375–3380.

34 Delmonico F. A report of the Amsterdam Forum on the Care of the Live Kidney Donor: data and medical guidelines. *Transplantation* 2005;79(6 Suppl):S53–S66.

35 Bright PD, Nutt J. The ethics surrounding HIV, kidney donation and patient confidentiality. *J Med Ethics* 2009;35(4):270–271.

36 United Kingdom Guidelines for Living Donor Kidney Transplantation. 2011. Available from http://www.bts.org.uk/transplantation/standards-and-guidelines/.

37 Textor SC, Taler SJ, Larson TS, Prieto M, Griffin M, Gloor J, *et al.* Blood pressure evaluation among older living kidney donors. *J Am Soc Nephrol* 2003;14(8):2159–2167.

38 Textor SC, Taler SJ, Driscoll N, Larson TS, Gloor J, Griffin M, *et al.* Blood pressure and renal function after kidney donation from hypertensive living donors. *Transplantation* 2004;78(2):276–282.

39 Torres VE, Offord KP, Anderson CF, Velosa JA, Frohnert PP, Donadio JV Jr,, *et al.* Blood pressure determinants in living-related renal allograft donors and their recipients. *Kidney Int* 1987;31(6):1383–1390.

40 Rule AD, Gussak HM, Pond GR, Bergstralh EJ, Stegall MD, Cosio FG, *et al.* Measured and estimated GFR in healthy potential kidney donors. *Am J Kidney Dis* 2004;43(1):112–119.

41 Bia MJ, Ramos EL, Danovitch GM, Gaston RS, Harmon WE, Leichtman AB, *et al.* Evaluation of living renal donors. *The current practice of US transplant centers. Transplantation* 1995;60(4):322–327.

42 Najarian JS, Chavers BM, McHugh LE, Matas AJ. 20 years or more of follow-up of living kidney donors. *Lancet* 1992;340(8823):807–810.

43 Matas AJ, Bartlett ST, Leichtman AB, Delmonico FL. Morbidity and mortality after living kidney donation, 1999–2001: survey of United States transplant centers. *Am J Transplant* 2003;3(7):830–834.

44 Schweitzer EJ, Wilson J, Jacobs S, Machan CH, Philosophe B, Farney A, *et al.* Increased rates of donation with laparoscopic donor nephrectomy. *Ann Surg* 2000;232(3):392–400.

45 Jacobs SC, Cho E, Foster C, Liao P, Bartlett ST. Laparoscopic donor nephrectomy: the University of Maryland 6-year experience. *J Urol* 2004;171(1):47–51.

46 Hadjianastassiou VG, Johnson RJ, Rudge CJ, Mamode N. 2509 living donor nephrectomies, morbidity and mortality, including the UK introduction of laparoscopic donor surgery. *Am J Transplant* 2007;7(11):2532–2537.

47 Narkun-Burgess DM, Nolan CR, Norman JE, Page WF, Miller PL, Meyer TW. Forty-five year follow-up after uninephrectomy. *Kidney Int* 1993;43(5): 1110–1115.

48 Ibrahim HN, Foley R, Tan L, Rogers T, Bailey RF, Guo H, *et al.* Long-term consequences of kidney donation. *N Engl J Med* 2009;360(5):459–469.

2 New Surgical Techniques in Transplantation

Adam D. Barlow and Michael L. Nicholson
Department of Transplant Surgery, University Hospitals of Leicester, UK

Introduction

Over the last decade, the major developments in renal-transplant-surgery techniques have been related to laparoscopic live-donor nephrectomy. However, in more recent years there have also been advances in surgical techniques in the recipient, particularly with regard to minimally invasive and robotic-assisted surgery.

This chapter discusses the various techniques for live-donor nephrectomy in detail, including the use of robotic-assisted surgery. Recent trends in the perioperative management of live donors are also examined. Finally, new techniques in recipient surgery are explored, including minimally invasive approaches, approaches to anastomosing multiple arteries, and the use of suture-free vascular anastomosis devices.

Live-donor nephrectomy: surgical techniques

Over recent years, living-donor renal transplantation has increasingly been used to offset the shortage of cadaveric kidneys. The surgical technique in the donor has evolved over this time from open nephrectomy via a flank incision with rib resection, through short-muscle-splitting incision without rib resection, to laparoscopic minimally invasive nephrectomy.

In the UK there has been a rapid increase in the number of transplant units performing laparoscopic donor nephrectomy. A recent survey conducted in Leicester has shown that over 80% of units now offer laparoscopic donor nephrectomy (unpublished data), as compared to 21% in 2002 [1]. This rise is based on good evidence of its benefit over traditional open surgery from randomized clinic trials and meta-analyses.

There are a number of different minimally invasive approaches, namely total laparoscopic donor nephrectomy (LDN), hand-assisted laparoscopic donor nephrectomy (HALDN), retroperitoneoscopic donor nephrectomy (RDN) and hand-assisted retroperitoneoscopic donor nephrectomy (HARDN).

Abdominal Organ Transplantation: State of the Art, First Edition.
Edited by Nizam Mamode and Raja Kandaswamy.
© 2013 Blackwell Publishing Ltd. Published 2013 by Blackwell Publishing Ltd.

Total laparoscopic donor nephrectomy

This procedure is performed with the donor in the lateral decubitus position, with the kidney to be removed uppermost. A 10–12 mm port is introduced either by direct vision or following Verress needle insufflation. Capnoperitoneum is established at 12–15 cm H_2O pressure and a 30° endoscope is introduced. Three to four additional 10–12 mm or 5 mm ports are inserted. The procedure begins by mobilizing and medially displacing the colon overlying the kidney; this dissection can be facilitated by the use of an ultrasonic or other electrosurgical dissector. The ureter and gonadal vein are then identified at the pelvic brim. The gonadal vein is followed superiorly to identify the renal vein. This is dissected free and its branches are controlled and divided. Our practice is to suture ligate the venous branches, utilizing laparoscopic knot-tying. This avoids metal clips adjacent to the renal vasculature, which might interfere with stapling of the vessels. The renal artery is identified posterior to the renal vein. On the left, this is dissected down to its origin at the aorta (see Figure 2.1) and on the right to the lateral border of the inferior vena cava or just beyond. If there are concerns regarding the length of the right renal artery, retrocaval dissection can be performed to allow division of the artery closer to its origin from the aorta. This is not for the fainthearted, however, as there is a risk of damage to posterior lumbar veins draining into the posterior cava. The resultant bleeding can be difficult or impossible to control laparoscopically, necessitating conversion to an open procedure. Following dissection of the renal vessels, the inferior, lateral, and superior attachments of the kidney are divided until the kidney is isolated on its vessels and ureter.

A 6 cm Pfannenstiel incision is then made, followed by a small incision in the peritoneum, and an endoscopic retrieval bag is introduced into the abdominal cavity. A purse-string suture is placed around the peritoneum

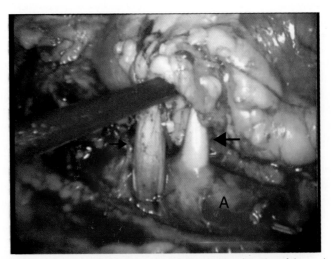

Figure 2.1 Intraoperative photograph during left LDN showing dissection of the renal vein (small arrow) and of the renal artery (large arrow) down to the aorta (A)

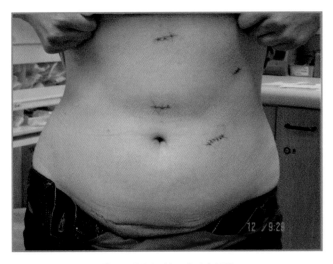

Figure 2.2 Incisions for left LDN

to maintain pneumoperitoneum. The ureter is first clipped and divided, and the renal vessels are then clipped or stapled. The kidney is placed in the bag and retrieved through the Pfannenstiel incision; it is then removed to the back table and flushed with preservative solution. Repeat laparoscopy is performed to ensure hemostasis prior to withdrawal of the ports and closure of the incisions. The resultant scars are shown in Figure 2.2.

The evidence

Alongside many nonrandomized studies, six randomized controlled trials [2–7] and two meta-analyses [8,9] have compared LDN with open techniques. Overall, these high-level studies have concluded that LDN results in significantly less analgesic requirements, shorter hospital stay (by 1.6 days, $p < 0.001$) and return to work (by 2.4 weeks, $p < 0.001$), and less chronic wound pain than open techniques, with similar complication rates [9]. However, this is at the expense of significantly longer operative times and, in some studies, increased first warm-ischemic time. Nevertheless, this does not appear to impact on graft outcome in the transplant recipients.

Hand-assisted laparoscopic donor nephrectomy

HALDN is performed in a similar fashion to LDN, but differs in that a hand port is placed at the extraction site. This can be done either at the beginning of the procedure or only for control of the vessels and extraction of the kidney. The hand port allows better tactile feedback, digital dissection, easier and quicker control of bleeding, and potentially quicker kidney extraction. Many surgeons feel HALDN improves the safety of LDN of donors, particularly when training or early in one's experience of LDN. Various incisions for the hand port have been described, including periumbilical, Pfannenstiel, and midline infraumbilical.

The evidence

The majority of (nonrandomized) studies comparing LDN with HALDN have concluded that HALDN results in shorter operating times, hospital stay, and first warm-ischemic time, with less blood loss [10–16]. However, the only randomized study comparing LDN with HALDN found that operating times were significantly longer in the HALDN group, with no difference in blood loss, warm-ischemic time, or length of hospital stay; this trial included only 40 patients, so it is difficult to draw firm conclusions [17]. There is also a study comparing right and left approaches after HALDN, showing no significant differences other than a shorter operating time for right kidneys [18].

Retroperitoneoscopic donor nephrectomy

This is performed with the patient in the lateral decubitus position. Following insertion of the initial port, the operating space is created by either digital dissection or using a balloon dilator. This space must extend to above the upper pole of the kidney and medially to the midline. The retroperitoneal space is maintained using CO_2 at a maximum pressure of 12 cm H_2O and a further two or three trocars are inserted. The retroperitoneal approach obviates any mobilization of the colon or spleen. The anteromedial portion of Gerota's fascia is opened and the upper pole of the kidney is dissected free. Attention is then turned to the renal vasculature, with the renal vein dissected free and its branches secured and divided. The artery is dissected down to the aorta on the left, or to the level of the inferior vena cava on the right. The ureter is then dissected down to the iliac vessels, and the lateral attachments of the kidney are divided. The ureter and vessels are divided and the kidney is removed via a preformed Pfannenstiel or lower midline incision.

The limited retroperitoneal space makes RDN potentially more technically challenging than LDN. This may be resolved somewhat by using a flexible laparoscope to improve visualization. In addition, tears in the peritoneum during dissection may result in escape of gas into the peritoneal cavity, reducing the retroperitoneal working space further. This can be remedied by placing a Verress needle into the peritoneal cavity to vent the escaped gas.

Nevertheless, the technical advantage of RDN is improved access to the retrorenal space, which particularly helps with managing posterior lumbar veins draining into the left renal vein and improves access to the retrocaval renal artery on the right. In addition, the peritoneal cavity is not breached, reducing the risk of bowel injury and intraabdominal adhesions.

The evidence

There have been no randomized controlled trials comparing RDN with either LDN or open techniques. The available case-control studies comparing RDN with open techniques have reported differing results in terms of operative time and warm-ischemic time, although RDN does appear to be associated with less postoperative pain [19,20]. The limited studies comparing RDN with LDN suggest equivalence between the two techniques in terms of postoperative pain, operative time, and warm-ischemic time [21,22].

As with LDN, hand-assisted RDN (HARDN) can also be performed, with the hand port placed at the Pfannenstiel extraction site. Again, HARDN has not been subjected to vigorous evaluation by randomized controlled trials, although recruitment to a multicenter study is currently taking place [23]. However, nonrandomized comparisons do appear to suggest that HARDN is significantly quicker than LDN [24,25].

Robotic-assisted laparoscopic donor nephrectomy

The use of robotic assistance has a number of advantages over conventional laparoscopic surgery, mainly related to visibility and dexterity. The instruments of the robotic devices have far greater degrees of movement and articulation than standard laparoscopic instruments and any hand tremor is filtered out by software. This allows more precise, delicate maneuvers and dissection. In addition, it enables restoration of the three-dimensional vision lost in standard laparoscopic surgery.

The technique for RALDN is as follows. The donor is placed in the lateral decubitus position. Four 10–12 mm laparoscopic ports are used: two for the robotic instruments, one for the laparoscope, and one for the assistant. Once the robotic instruments are docked as shown in Figure 2.3, the surgeon is seated at the remote console. The assistant remains at the operating table and is responsible for instrument exchanges, suction-irrigation, clip application, and insertion or extraction of the endoscopic retrieval bag. The dissection and extraction of the kidney proceeds as described for LDN.

The evidence

The first report of RALDN was published in 2002 from the University of Illinois at Chicago, describing 10 successful cases [26]. Since then, a number of other centers have reported their experience. Hubert *et al.* described

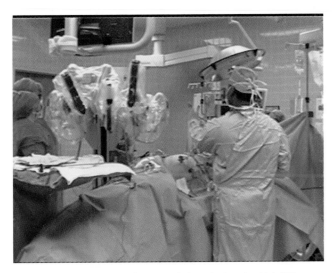

Figure 2.3 Da Vinci robot in use during robotic-assisted left LDN

RALDN in 38 donors, with a mean operating time of 181 minutes, no conversions, and no intraoperative complications [27]. The University of Illinois at Chicago has reported its further experience with 209 left RALDNs [28]. These included 61 patients with multiple renal vessels requiring back-table reconstruction. Mean operating time was 152 minutes, delayed graft function was 0%, open conversion for bleeding was necessary in four patients (2%), and mean length of stay for the donor was 2 days.

However, there are no randomized controlled trials of RALDN, and currently there is no clear evidence of any clinical benefit from robotic-assisted procurement.

The greatest barrier to RALDN is currently the cost of purchasing and maintaining the robotic equipment. The only commercial robotic-surgery system currently available is the da Vinci Surgical System (Intuitive Surgical Inc., Sunnyvale, CA, USA) (Figure 2.3), which has a cost of over US$1.25 million. Unless this figure drops dramatically, this technology is going to be unavailable to the vast majority of transplant centers, particularly without evidence of resounding clinical or cost benefits over conventional laparoscopic donor nephrectomy.

Single-port donor nephrectomy

Laparoendoscopic single-site (LESS) surgery is a recent development in minimally invasive surgery. This technique employs a single-access multi-channel port such as the TriPort (Olympus Keymed, Southend-on-Sea, UK) or SILS port (Covidien, Dublin, Ireland). These ports are inserted through a 2–3 cm Pfannenstiel or vertical intraumbilical incision and allow simultaneous passage of a laparoscope and two instruments. The use of curved and articulating laparoscopic instruments prevents clashing of instruments and restores some of the triangulation lost due to the close insertion points.

Intraabdominally, the LESS LDN mirrors the conventional LDN. The kidney is extracted in an endobag through an extension of the LESS incision.

The evidence

To date, at least seven centers have reported their experience of LESS surgery for donor nephrectomy. These have confirmed the feasibility of the technique. Of the two studies comparing LESS with conventional LDN, one reports no difference between the groups in terms of operative time, warm-ischemic time, analgesia requirements, and pain scores, while the other shows a significantly quicker return to work and full physical recovery in the LESS group [29,30]. A recent randomized controlled trial comparing LESS with conventional LDN in 50 patients found LESS to result in significantly longer warm-ischemic times (5 versus 7 minutes, $p < 0.0001$) but slightly shorter hospital stay (4.6 versus 3.9 days, $p = 0.003$). The estimated glomerular filtration rate at 1 year was comparable between the groups [31].

Transvaginal extraction of the kidney

There have been two recent reports of laparoscopic donor nephrectomy with transvaginal extraction of the kidney. This builds on the concept of natural-orifice transluminal surgery (NOTES), whereby surgery is performed through natural orifices (e.g. vagina, mouth, and rectum), thereby eliminating scars and potentially reducing pain, due to the differing innervation of internal organs as compared to the abdominal wall.

Transvaginal extraction of the kidney following laparoscopic right donor nephrectomy [32] and robotic-assisted laparoscopic left donor nephrectomy [33] have been reported, the former in a patient who had previously undergone laparoscopic hysterectomy. Interestingly, neither patient required postoperative parenteral analgesia.

This technique is obviously in its infancy and requires further evaluation. It inherently excludes male patients and the acceptability to young nulliparious women is unanswered. It will be interesting to see if a pure transvaginal NOTES approach to donor nephrectomy becomes feasible in the future.

Mini-incision donor nephrectomy

Rather than pursuing the laparoscopic route, some centers have taken the approach of refining the open technique to allow much smaller incisions. A number of techniques of so-called mini-incision donor nephrectomy (MIDN) have been described. In general, these involve a transverse incision just anterior to the 11th rib, which is not resected. This incision is around 8 cm in length, with one center reporting a final median length of incision of 6.8 cm [34]. The abdominal-wall muscles are split rather than cut. Exposure through these small incisions can be facilitated by the use of specialized retractors such as the Omnitract (Omnitract Surgical, St Paul, MN, USA), Hakim lighted retractor (Bolton Surgical, Sheffield, UK), or Deaver retractors. In addition, with limited access, control of the renal vessel may be easier using articulating linear vascular staplers rather than conventional vascular clamps and suturing.

The evidence

A recent meta-analysis comparing MIDN with standard open donor nephrectomy showed no significant differences in operative time, warm ischemia, or blood loss. However, hospital stay and return to work were significantly shorter for MIDN, and analgesia requirements and overall complications were also significantly less [8]. When comparing MIDN with LDN, the same study found significantly shorter operative and warm-ischemic times, but significantly higher analgesia requirements, for MIDN [6]. These results should be treated with caution, as of the nine studies included in the meta-analysis, only one was a randomized controlled trial. That study, which compared LDN with MIDN, concluded that LDN resulted in significantly longer operating and warm-ischemia times, but significantly less morphine use and a significantly shorter hospital stay. In addition, physical fatigue and physical function were significantly improved at 1 year following LDN [3]. A cost-effectiveness analysis of the same study showed that LDN was more cost-effective [35].

Perioperative management of the live donor

During the initial development of laparoscopic donor nephrectomy, concerns were raised about the detrimental effects to the kidney of the increased abdominal pressure associated with prolonged capnoperitoneum. Certainly, animal studies have shown clear decreases in renal blood flow and urine output during capnoperitoneum [36]. As such, aggressive pre- and periop- erative fluid resuscitation was recommended to optimize cardiac preload and counter these detrimental effects [37]. However, this approach is not without drawbacks, and unilateral pulmonary edema following laparoscopic donor nephrectomy has been reported by a number of centers.

Recent work on intraoperative fluid management in LDN has challenged the dogma of aggressive fluid hydration for all. A prospective compar- ison of intraoperative fluid-load (>10 ml/kg/hour) versus fluid-restrict (<10 ml/kg/hour) regimens for LDN in 52 patients showed that while fluid restriction resulted in a lower intraoperative urine output, there were no significant differences in renal function in either the donor or the recipient up to 12 months following surgery [38]. A further small randomized study showed that while aggressive fluid management significantly increased stroke volume, there was no significant difference in creatinine clearance from day 2 postoperatively [39], although this may be a reflection of the sample size.

Another approach to counteracting intraoperative oliguria during laparo- scopic donor nephrectomy is the use of renal-dose dopamine. One retrospective study comparing perioperative mannitol in open donor nephrectomy with mannitol and dopamine in LDN showed significantly greater operative urine output in the latter group, but no differences in early graft function [40]. A further retrospective study comparing dopamine infusion in LDN with standard management found no beneficial effects on renal function to either donor or recipient [41]. Therefore, there is no evidence of a benefit of dopamine in the perioperative management of living kidney donors.

In an effort to optimize perioperative fluid management in live-donor nephrectomy, a number of centers, ours included, have adopted esophageal Doppler as a noninvasive measure of cardiac preload. This technique involves the insertion of a flexible probe into the distal esophagus to measure blood-flow velocity in the descending aorta. Cardiac output is estimated by multiplying the blood-flow velocity by cross-sectional area of the aorta at the measured point. One study comparing central venous pressure (CVP) monitoring with esophageal Doppler monitoring during laparoscopic donor nephrectomy found that while lateral positioning and pneumoperitoneum significantly increased CVP, no changes in cardiac output, as estimated by esophageal Doppler, were seen [42]. The authors remark that they decreased the total fluid administered during LDN as they began to use the esophageal Doppler. Although this is of interest, further studies are required to elucidate the true benefit of esophageal Doppler monitoring during LDN.

There are other noninvasive methods of cardiac-output monitoring which may be applicable to LDN. Lithium-dilution cardiac output (LiDCO) involves intravascular injection of a small dose of lithium chloride via a peripheral line. The resulting lithium concentration–time curve is recorded by withdrawing blood through a disposable sensor attached to the patient's arterial line, and the cardiac output is derived mathematically from this. As yet, no studies have been conducted using LiDCO for hemodynamic optimization during donor nephrectomy.

Surgical advances in renal-transplantation techniques

The fundamental surgical technique for implanting a renal transplant has changed little since Alexis Carrel first developed a successful method for vascular anastomosis in the early 1900s. However, in recent years there has been a move to develop minimally invasive techniques. In addition, as the number of live-donor kidneys retrieved with multiple arteries has increased, techniques for anastomosing multiple arteries have developed.

Minimally invasive renal transplantation

Traditionally, kidney transplantation has been performed through a large incision approximately 20 cm long, dividing all muscle layers and with wide exposure of the iliac vessels. Some centers worldwide have endeavored to develop minimally invasive techniques, limiting the incision to less than 10 cm.

Oyen et al. have reported minimally invasive kidney transplantation (MIKT) in 21 patients [43]. A 7–9 cm transverse incision is made 3–5 cm above the inguinal ligament, with the medial end 2–3 cm from the midline. The conjoint tendon is divided, but all other muscle layers are split. Exposure is facilitated by the Omnitract system. A lateral retroperitoneal pouch is created and the kidney is placed within it. All three anastomoses are performed with the kidney in this final position. This necessitates suturing the posterior wall of the vessels from within the vessel. Ureteric reimplantation is performed using the Lich–Gregoir extravesical technique with no stent. In comparison with a matched group undergoing conventional kidney transplantation, this study found MIKT to be significantly quicker and to result in a shorter hospital stay, with no difference in graft function.

In addition, Mun et al. have reported a series of MIKTs with video assistance [44]. Their technique is as follows. Preoperative ultrasound is used to mark the course of the external iliac vessels, the contour of the urinary bladder, and the lateral margin of the rectus muscle. A 7–8 cm incision is made from the line of the iliac vessels to the lateral edge of the urinary bladder. The abdominal-wall musculature is divided and a laparoscopic balloon dilator is used to develop a retroperitoneal space for the transplant kidney. Following dissection of the iliac vessels, the vascular anastomoses are performed either with the kidney placed just above the vessels or with it in the retroperitoneal pouch. During vascular anastomosis, a laparoscope is used to provide further illumination and better visualization of the surgical field for the assistant. Ureteric anastomosis is performed using an extravesicular technique. In comparison with an unmatched group undergoing conventional kidney transplantation, MIKT resulted in significantly less postoperative pain and opiate use, along with significantly quicker return to work and resumption of normal activities. There was no difference in hospital stay or graft function between the groups.

Despite the findings of these studies, there are some concerns with MIKT. Back-table preparation of the kidney must be meticulous, particularly with respect to hemostasis, as access to control hilar bleeding is limited. A short renal vein also makes MIKT either challenging or impossible, necessitating back-bench reconstruction with caval tube or saphenous vein. Furthermore, MIKT is not suitable for recipients with significantly raised body mass index (BMI). Further study in the form of a randomized controlled trial comparing MIKT with conventional kidney transplantation is required to fully elucidate the benefits.

Laparoscopic renal transplantation

The feasibility of laparoscopic renal transplantation was first established in 2001 using a pig autotransplantation model [45]. However, of concern were the mean operating time of over 6 hours and the mean anastomosis time of 64 minutes.

It took a further 9 years before the first report of laparoscopic kidney transplantation in a human was published [46]. This first case was performed without robotic assistance. More recently, two further reports of robotic-assisted renal transplantation, one from the University of Illinois at Chicago, USA [47], and one from the University of Pisa, Italy [48], have been published. All three transplants were implanted on to the recipient's right iliac vessels via a transabdominal approach. The kidneys were introduced into the abdomen through a hand port placed in either a Pfannenstiel or a midline incision. All three transplants functioned immediately.

Although laparoscopic renal transplantation can be done, the question remains should it be done? In all of the above reports, warm-ischemic time was between 50 and 60 minutes. Although this did not have adverse effects in these cases, it may have an effect on more borderline kidney grafts, such as those from non-heart-beating donors. Given the scarcity of donor kidneys, there would have to be very clear evidence of a benefit of laparoscopic kidney transplantation to justify the increased risk of graft failure or dysfunction.

Implantation of renal grafts with multiple vessels

There are a number of techniques available for anastomosing multiple renal arteries, as demonstrated in Figure 2.4. Two arteries may be joined together at their orifices to form a single trunk for anastomosis, for example (Figure 2.4a). A smaller polar artery may be anastomosed end-to-side to a larger renal artery (Figure 2.4b). Alternatively, a lower-polar artery may be anastomosed end-to-end to the inferior epigastric artery, with the main renal artery anastomosed to the iliac system (Figure 2.4c).

A further technique is to dissect out the internal iliac artery to the point where it branches. These separate lumens can then be used to anastomose separate renal arteries (Figure 2.4d). We have recently reported a refinement of this technique whereby the main trunk of the recipient internal artery is divided and the distal artery explanted [49]. This allows careful back-bench

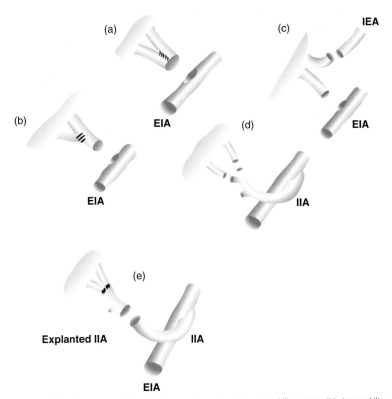

Figure 2.4 Methods of anastomosis for multiple renal arteries. EIA, external iliac artery; IIA, internal iliac artery; IEA, inferior epigastric artery

anastomosis of multiple renal arteries to the internal iliac artery, which can be aided by the use of pediatric feeding tubes (see Figure 2.5), without concerns over warm ischemia. Once completed, the explanted distal iliac artery is reanastomosed end-to-end to its proximal portion (Figure 2.4e). This large single anastomosis can be performed more quickly than the multiple small anastomoses, limiting warm-ischemic time.

Sutureless vascular anastomosis

Although suturing remains the standard technique, the quest for simpler, faster, and less technically demanding methods of performing vascular anastomosis has led to the development of a number of alternative sutureless techniques. Those currently available commercially include rings, clips, and stents.

The Unilink ring system (3M, St Paul, MN, USA) was first introduced in 1986. It consists of two polyethylene rings: one with stainless steel pins and the other with corresponding holes. The vessel ends are inserted over the rings, which are approximated using a special device. There are a number of successful reports of the use of this system for microvascular anastomosis of free flaps for head and neck reconstruction [50]. The system

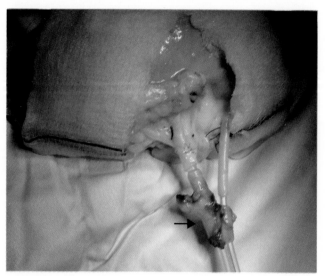

Figure 2.5 Explanted internal iliac artery (arrow) being used to transplant a kidney with multiple vessels

seems best suited to end-to-end anastomosis of nonatherosclerotic vessels with minimal size discrepancy. Although the use of the Unilink system has not been reported in renal transplantation, use of a similar metal-ring pin stapler in 36 renal-transplant recipients has been published [51]. This showed mechanical anastomosis to be quicker than the conventional suturing technique, with no technical failures.

The only commercially available clip system for vascular anastomosis is the VCS clip applier system (Autosuture, Norwalk, CT, USA). This instrument allows the application of individual small titanium clips to everted vessel edges. Studies of its use in a variety of settings, including arteriovenous fistula formation, coronary-artery bypass grafting, and free tissue transfer, have demonstrated advantages including a reduced anastomotic time and a higher patency rate. Two centers have reported their experience of the VCS for vascular anastomosis in renal transplant in a combined total of 36 patients [52,53]. In one of these studies, this technique was shown to be quicker than sutured anastomosis [52].

Overall, the experience of sutureless vascular anastomosis in renal transplantation is very limited. However, the VCS clip applier, in particular, does seem worthy of further study in the form of a randomized controlled trial comparing it with sutured anastomosis.

Conclusion

Laparoscopic donor nephrectomy has clear benefits over conventional surgery and should be the technique of choice. There are particular advantages to each laparoscopic technique, and debate continues over the most beneficial. There is no clear evidence of benefit from robotic assistance. Future developments may include single-port and natural-orifice laparoscopic surgery. Mini-incision nephrectomy may be better than conventional open surgery but inferior to laparoscopic surgery.

Advances have been made in the introduction of minimally invasive recipient surgery, including laparoscopic, robotic, and sutureless surgery. Further refinements of these techniques and large trials are awaited with interest.

References

1 Brook NR, Nicholson ML. An audit over 2 years' practice of open and laparoscopic live-donor nephrectomy at renal transplant centres in the UK and Ireland. *BJU Int* 2004;93(7):1027–1031.

2 Nicholson ML, Kaushik M, Lewis GR, Brook NR, Bagul A, Kay MD, *et al.* Randomized clinical trial of laparoscopic versus open donor nephrectomy. *Br J Surg* 2010;97(1):21–28.

3 Kok NF, Lind MY, Hansson BM, Pilzecker D, Mertens zur Borg IR, Knipscheer BC, *et al.* Comparison of laparoscopic and mini incision open donor nephrectomy: single blind, randomised controlled clinical trial. *BMJ* 2006;333(7561):221.

4 Oyen O, Andersen M, Mathisen L, Kvarstein G, Edwin B, Line PD, *et al.* Laparoscopic versus open living-donor nephrectomy: experiences from a prospective, randomized, single-center study focusing on donor safety. *Transplantation* 2005;79(9):1236–1240.

5 Simforoosh N, Basiri A, Tabibi A, Shakhssalim N, Hosseini Moghaddam SM. Comparison of laparoscopic and open donor nephrectomy: a randomized controlled trial. *BJU Int* 2005;95(6):851–855.

6 Wolf JS Jr,, Merion RM, Leichtman AB, Campbell DA Jr,, Magee JC, Punch JD, Turcotte JG, Konnak JW. Randomized controlled trial of hand-assisted laparoscopic versus open surgical live donor nephrectomy. *Transplantation* 2001;72:284–290.

7 Basiri A, Simforoosh N, Heidari M, Moghaddam SM, Otookesh H. Laparoscopic v open donor nephrectomy for pediatric kidney recipients: preliminary report of a randomized controlled trial. *J Endourol* 2007;21(9):1033–1036.

8 Antcliffe D, Nanidis TG, Darzi AW, Tekkis PP, Papalois VE. A meta-analysis of mini-open versus standard open and laparoscopic living donor nephrectomy. *Transpl Int* 2009;22(4):463–474.

9 Nanidis TG, Antcliffe D, Kokkinos C, Borysiewicz CA, Darzi AW, Tekkis PP, *et al.* Laparoscopic versus open live donor nephrectomy in renal transplantation: a meta-analysis. *Ann Surg* 2008;247(1):58–70.

10 El-Galley R, Hood N, Young CJ, Deierhoi M, Urban DA. Donor nephrectomy: a comparison of techniques and results of open, hand assisted and full laparoscopic nephrectomy. *J Urol* 2004;171(1):40–43.

11 Mateo RB, Sher L, Jabbour N, Singh G, Chan L, Selby RR, *et al.* Comparison of outcomes in noncomplicated and in higher-risk donors after standard versus hand-assisted laparoscopic nephrectomy. *Am Surg* 2003;69(9):771–778.

12 Gershbein AB, Fuchs GJ. Hand-assisted and conventional laparoscopic live donor nephrectomy: a comparison of two contemporary techniques. *J Endourol* 2002;16(7):509–513.

13 Lindstrom P, Haggman M, Wadstrom J. Hand-assisted laparoscopic surgery (HALS) for live donor nephrectomy is more time- and cost-effective than standard laparoscopic nephrectomy. *Surg Endosc* 2002;16(3):422–425.

14 Velidedeoglu E, Williams N, Brayman KL, Desai NM, Campos L, Palanjian M, *et al.* Comparison of open, laparoscopic, and hand-assisted approaches to live-donor nephrectomy. *Transplantation* 2002;74(2):169–172.

15 Buell JF, Hanaway MJ, Potter SR, Cronin DC, Yoshida A, Munda R, *et al.* Hand-assisted laparoscopic living-donor nephrectomy as an alternative to traditional laparoscopic living-donor nephrectomy. *Am J Transplant* 2002;2(10):983–988.

16 Ruiz-Deya G, Cheng S, Palmer E, Thomas R, Slakey D. Open donor, laparoscopic donor and hand assisted laparoscopic donor nephrectomy: a comparison of outcomes. *J Urol* 2001;166(4):1270–1273, disc. 1273–1274.

17 Bargman V, Sundaram CP, Bernie J, Goggins W. Randomized trial of laparoscopic donor nephrectomy with and without hand assistance. *J Endourol* 2006;20(10):717–722.

18 Minnee RC, Bemelman WA, Maartense S, Bemelman FJ, Gouma DJ, Idu MM. Left or right kidney in hand-assisted donor nephrectomy? A randomized controlled trial. *Transplantation* 2008;85(2):203–208.

19 Bachmann A, Wolff T, Ruszat R, Giannini O, Dickenmann M, Gurke L, *et al.* Retroperitoneoscopic donor nephrectomy: a retrospective, non-randomized comparison of early complications, donor and recipient outcome with the standard open approach. *Eur Urol* 2005;48(1):90–96, disc. 96.

20 Bachmann A, Dickenmann M, Gurke L, Giannini O, Langer I, Gasser TC, *et al.* Retroperitoneoscopic living donor nephrectomy: a retrospective comparison to the open approach. *Transplantation* 2004;78(1):168–171.

21 Buell JF, Abreu SC, Hanaway MJ, Ng CS, Kaouk JH, Clippard M, *et al.* Right donor nephrectomy: a comparison of hand-assisted transperitoneal and retroperitoneal laparoscopic approaches. *Transplantation* 2004;77(4):521–525.

22 Ng CS, Abreu SC, Abou El-Fettouh HI, Kaouk JH, Desai MM, Goldfarb DA, *et al.* Right retroperitoneal versus left transperitoneal laparoscopic live donor nephrectomy. *Urology* 2004;63(5):857–861.

23 Dols LF, Kok NF, Terkivatan T, Tran TC, d'Ancona FC, Langenhuijsen JF, *et al.* Hand-assisted retroperitoneoscopic versus standard laparoscopic donor nephrectomy: HARP-trial. *BMC Surg* 2010;10:11.

24 Gjertsen H, Sandberg AK, Wadstrom J, Tyden G, Ericzon BG. Introduction of hand-assisted retroperitoneoscopic living donor nephrectomy at Karolinska University Hospital Huddinge. *Transplant Proc* 2006;38(8):2644–2645.

25 Sundqvist P, Feuk U, Haggman M, Persson AE, Stridsberg M, Wadstrom J. Hand-assisted retroperitoneoscopic live donor nephrectomy in comparison to open and laparoscopic procedures: a prospective study on donor morbidity and kidney function. *Transplantation* 2004;78(1):147–153.

26 Horgan S, Vanuno D, Sileri P, Cicalese L, Benedetti E. Robotic-assisted laparoscopic donor nephrectomy for kidney transplantation. *Transplantation* 2002;73(9):1474–1479.

27 Hubert J, Renoult E, Mourey E, Frimat L, Cormier L, Kessler M. Complete robotic-assistance during laparoscopic living donor nephrectomies: an evaluation of 38 procedures at a single site. *Int J Urol* 2007;14(11):986–989.

28 Gorodner V, Horgan S, Galvani C, Manzelli A, Oberholzer J, Sankary H, *et al.* Routine left robotic-assisted laparoscopic donor nephrectomy is safe and effective regardless of the presence of vascular anomalies. *Transpl Int* 2006;19(8):636–640.

29 Andonian S, Rais-Bahrami S, Atalla MA, Herati AS, Richstone L, Kavoussi LR. Laparoendoscopic single-site Pfannenstiel versus standard laparoscopic donor nephrectomy. *J Endourol* 2010;24(3):429–432.

30 Canes D, Berger A, Aron M, Brandina R, Goldfarb DA, Shoskes D, *et al.* Laparo-endoscopic single site (LESS) versus standard laparoscopic left donor nephrectomy: matched-pair comparison. *Eur Urol* 2010;57(1):95–101.

31 Kurien A, Rajapurkar S, Sinha L, Mishra S, Ganpule A, Muthu V, *et al.* Standard laparoscopic donor nephrectomy versus laparoendoscopic single-site donor nephrectomy: a randomized comparative study. *J Endourol* 2011;25(3):365–370.

32 Allaf ME, Singer A, Shen W, Green I, Womer K, Segev DL, *et al.* Laparoscopic live donor nephrectomy with vaginal extraction: initial report. *Am J Transplant* 2010;10(6):1473–1477.

33 Pietrabissa A, Abelli M, Spinillo A, Alessiani M, Zonta S, Ticozzelli E, *et al.* Robotic-assisted laparoscopic donor nephrectomy with transvaginal extraction of the kidney. *Am J Transplant* 2010;10(12):2708–2711.

34 Hakim N, Aboutaleb E, Syed A, Rajagopal P, Herbert P, Canelo R, *et al.* A fast and safe living donor "finger-assisted" nephrectomy technique: results of 359 cases. *Transplant Proc* 2010;42(1):165–170.

35 Cost effectiveness of laparoscopic versus mini-incision open donor nephrectomy: a randomized study. Kok NF, Adang EM, Hansson BM, Dooper IM, Weimar W, van der Wilt GJ, Ijzermans JN. *Transplantation.* 2007;83(12):1582–1587.

36 London ET, Ho HS, Neuhaus AM, Wolfe BM, Rudich SM, Perez RV. Effect of intravascular volume expansion on renal function during prolonged CO2 pneumoperitoneum. *Ann Surg* 2000;231(2):195–201.

37 Flowers JL, Jacobs S, Cho E, Morton A, Rosenberger WF, Evans D, *et al.* Comparison of open and laparoscopic live donor nephrectomy. *Ann Surg* 1997;226(4):483–489, disc. 489–490.

38 Bergman S, Feldman LS, Carli F, Anidjar M, Vassiliou MC, Andrew CG, *et al.* Intraoperative fluid management in laparoscopic live-donor nephrectomy: challenging the dogma. *Surg Endosc* 2004;18(11):1625–1630.

39 Mertens zur Borg IR, Di Biase M, Verbrugge S, Ijzermans JN, Gommers D. Comparison of three perioperative fluid regimes for laparoscopic donor nephrectomy: a prospective randomized dose-finding study. *Surg Endosc* 2008;22(1):146–150.

40 Bolte SL, Chin LT, Moon TD, D'Alessandro AM, Nakada SY, Becker YT, *et al.* Maintaining urine production and early allograft function during laparoscopic donor nephrectomy. *Urology* 2006;68(4):747–750.

41 O'Dair J, Evans L, Rigg KM, Shehata M. Routine use of renal-dose dopamine during living donor nephrectomy has no beneficial effect to either donor or recipient. *Transplant Proc* 2005;37(2):637–639.

42 Feldman LS, Anidjar M, Metrakos P, Stanbridge D, Fried GM, Carli F. Optimization of cardiac preload during laparoscopic donor nephrectomy: a preliminary study of central venous pressure versus esophageal Doppler monitoring. *Surg Endosc* 2004;18(3):412–416.

43 Oyen O, Scholz T, Hartmann A, Pfeffer P. Minimally invasive kidney transplantation: the first experience. *Transplant Proc* 2006;38(9):2798–2802.

44 Mun SP, Chang JH, Kim KJ, Jeong GA, Cheon MW, Ahn YJ, *et al.* Minimally invasive video-assisted kidney transplantation (MIVAKT). *J Surg Res* 2007;141(2):204–210.

45 Meraney AM, Gill IS, Kaouk JH, Skacel M, Sung GT. Laparoscopic renal autotransplantation. *J Endourol* 2001;15(2):143–149.

46 Rosales A, Salvador JT, Urdaneta G, Patino D, Montlleo M, Esquena S, *et al.* Laparoscopic kidney transplantation. *Eur Urol* 2010;57(1):164–167.

47 Giulianotti P, Gorodner V, Sbrana F, Tzvetanov I, Jeon H, Bianco F, *et al.* Robotic transabdominal kidney transplantation in a morbidly obese patient. *Am J Transplant* 2010;10(6):1478–1482.

48 Boggi U, Vistoli F, Signori S, D'Imporzano S, Amorese G, Consani G, *et al.* Robotic renal transplantation: first European case. *Transpl Int* 2011;24(2):213–218.

49 Firmin LC, Nicholson ML. The use of explanted internal iliac artery grafts in renal transplants with multiple arteries. *Transplantation* 2010 Mar 27;89(6):766–767.

50 Chernichenko N, Ross DA, Shin J, Chow JY, Sasaki CT, Ariyan S. Arterial coupling for microvascular free tissue transfer. *Otolaryngol Head Neck Surg* 2008;138(5):614–618.

51 Ye G, Mo HG, Wang ZH, Yi SH, Wang XW, Zhang YF. Arterial anastomosis without sutures using ring pin stapler for clinical renal transplantation: comparison with suture anastomosis. *J Urol* 2006;175(2):636–640, disc. 640.

52 Al-Habash MM, Al-Shaer MB. Use of vascular clipping system in kidney transplantation in syria: a study of 30 cases. *Saudi J Kidney Dis Transpl* 2002;13(1):35–39.

53 Papalois VE, Romagnoli J, Hakim NS. Use of vascular closure staples in vascular access for dialysis, kidney and pancreas transplantation. *Int Surg* 1998;83(2):177–180.

3 Living-donor Liver Transplantation

Abhideep Chaudhary and Abhinav Humar

Department of Surgery, University of Pittsburgh, Medical Center (UPMC), USA

History

Liver transplantation has been the standard of care for almost 3 decades for patients with end-stage liver disease. The scarcity of donor organs is the major limiting factor in liver transplantation. Over 16 000 people are now waiting for a liver transplant in the USA, but only about 6000 transplants are performed every year. Roughly 10–15% of the candidates each year die of their liver disease before having the chance to undergo a transplant [1]. For those who do end up receiving a transplant from a deceased donor, the waiting time can be significant, resulting in severe debilitation. With a living-donor liver transplant (LDLT), this waiting time can be reduced, allowing the transplant to be performed before the recipient's health deteriorates further. In areas of the world where deceased-donor transplants are not performed, due to nonexistent deceased-donor graft donation, the advantages of LDLT are even more obvious. LDLT evolved from experience gained from in situ deceased-donor hepatectomy with reduced-size and split grafts, an idea first proposed by Smith in 1969 [2].

The first LDLT was from an adult to a child using the left lobe of the liver and was performed by Raia in Brazil in 1988, but the recipient did not survive [3]. The first successful adult-to-child LDLT was performed in Australia in 1989 by Russel Strong [4]. The Chicago Group, led by Broelsch, developed the first adult-to-child LDLT program in the USA [5]. LDLT started growing rapidly following its debut and living donation of the lateral segment of the left lobe of the liver has become highly successful in pediatric transplantation. With the success of LDLT in pediatric recipients, left-lobe LDLT was extended to adults; the first such transplant was reported by Makuuchi *et al.*, but the overall success was marred by the donor organ being small for the recipient's size [6]. The Kyoto Group in 1994 performed the first right-liver graft in a child, as the donor left-lobe arterial supply was unfavorable [7]. Fan and his team, at the University of Hong Kong, first performed adult-to-adult LDLT using the right hemiliver in 1996, with

Abdominal Organ Transplantation: State of the Art, First Edition.
Edited by Nizam Mamode and Raja Kandaswamy.
© 2013 Blackwell Publishing Ltd. Published 2013 by Blackwell Publishing Ltd.

a favorable outcome [8]. Since that time, many centers have adopted the procedure, not only in Asia but in other parts of the world as well. The first adult LDLT in the USA utilizing the right lobe was reported by Wachs *et al.* in 1998 [9].

In the present-day scenario, LDLT accounts for almost 4% of all liver transplantation in the USA [1] and a significantly higher percentage in Asia and other parts of the world. LDLT has continued to evolve in recent years, leading to increased donor safety and better public acceptance. Short-term results and outcomes have become well described with this procedure, but longer-term results, both in donors and in recipients, need to be better defined.

Donor evaluation

The evaluation of individuals who present as possible liver donors is a crucial part of the LDLT process. A complete and thorough evaluation is important in minimizing the risks of the procedure for the potential donor and in optimizing donor safety—the underlying principle of any living-donor procedure [10]. The pre-donation evaluation of the potential donor, and characterization of the subsequent liver graft that they may yield, is also critical in ensuring a successful outcome for the recipient. The evaluation process may vary between donors, depending on whether the recipient is an adult or a pediatric patient, the size of the planned liver resection, and the individual center's preference. But the major steps of the process remain basically the same, and can be divided into three major parts: (i) medical evaluation, (ii) surgical and radiological evaluation, and (iii) psychosocial evaluation. The potential donor should satisfy each of the three parts of this evaluation process before being considered acceptable. The evaluation process should, at the same time as being complete, not be overly cumbersome for the donor. It should be streamlined and efficient, and invasive and costly tests should be minimized and reserved for the later part of the evaluation, after the donor has passed through the initial screening process. Members of multiple teams need to be involved in the evaluation process. These should include a hepatologist, a surgeon, a psychologist, a social worker, and a transplant coordinator.

Medical evaluation

The medical evaluation of the potential donor has several goals and attempts to answer several important questions. One essential goal is to ensure that the donor does not have underlying medical problems that would significantly increase the risk associated with a general anesthetic and a major intra-abdominal procedure. This part of the evaluation is not too dissimilar from the evaluation for any individual undergoing a major general surgical procedure. The other important part of the medical evaluation serves to identify and exclude any possibility of chronic liver disease or liver dysfunction in the potential donor. This includes screening for viral pathogens that might impact on the donor's liver function, or could potentially be significantly harmful when transmitted to the recipient.

The most useful part of the medical evaluation is the initial screening history—this may be performed by an experienced transplant coordinator (a phone interview is adequate), or else the donor can be asked to fill out a one- or two-page information sheet. Questions regarding age, height, weight, blood type (if known), past and current medical, surgical, or psychosocial problems (including a history of alcohol use), and current medication use are very helpful. Donors with a significant past medical history, obese donors, and those with significant comorbidities can be excluded with the screening history, thus avoiding a detailed and expensive evaluation process. Age is an important variable to determine at the initial screening and potential donors falling outside the center's accepted age criteria can be excluded early. There are insufficient live-donor liver data at present to define an upper age limit for donation. Many centers have chosen 55, but potential donors have been considered by some centers up to the age of 60. Based upon data from the general surgical literature and experimental regeneration data, the limit of 60 has been considered appropriate. The lower limit of age for donation is determined by the ability to give legal consent.

After the initial screening history, basic screening labs should be performed—all of these can be performed at the laboratory that is physically closest to the potential donor. Tests to be included are complete blood count, serum electrolyte levels, liver-function tests, lipid profile, and blood type [11]. Based on the results of the screening history and screening labs, the potential donor can be brought into the transplant center for a more thorough evaluation.

The next part of the evaluation begins with a careful history and physical examination by a physician. Some feel that this should be performed by a physician who is not directly involved with the transplant team, and can therefore provide an unbiased opinion, without knowledge of the potential recipient. Individuals identified with significant underlying disorders of the cardiac, respiratory, or renal systems should be excluded from donation. Individuals with underlying risk factors for specific organ systems (e.g. age >40 and positive family history for cardiac disease) may require specialist consultation and more specific tests (e.g. echocardiogram or stress test). More detailed laboratory tests should also be performed during this part of the evaluation, including detailed viral serological evaluation (Hep C, Hep B, CMV, EBV, and HIV), screening for thrombophilia disorders (protein C, protein S, antithrombin III, factor V Leiden mutation, prothrombin mutation, and cardiolipin/antiphospholipids antibodies), and tests to exclude underlying chronic liver diseases (serum transferrin saturation, ferritin, α 1-antitrypsin antinuclear antibody, smooth-muscle antibody, and antimitochondrial antibody). Other tests that should be performed at this initial visit include electrocardiography, chest radiography, and pulmonary-function tests (if there is a history of smoking or asthma). Additional laboratory tests and imaging studies may be needed based on abnormalities identified in the history and the physical.

Special issues in the medical evaluation
Donor obesity
Body mass index (BMI) is a useful parameter to measure in the donor as a number of studies have shown a good correlation between obesity (BMI $>28\,kg/m^2$) and hepatic steatosis. One study suggested that 78% of potential donors with a BMI $>28\,kg/m^2$ had $>10\%$ steatosis on liver biopsy [12]. However, not all studies have shown this degree of correlation, and mild degrees of obesity may not be associated with significant steatosis in many cases. In such cases, a more direct evaluation of the liver parenchyma, usually with a liver biopsy, may be necessary to rule out the possibility of hepatic steatosis.

An additional problem with the use of obese donors is the potential for increased surgical risk in the donor. Studies from the general surgery literature suggest an increased incidence of surgical complications such as bleeding and wound problems in obese individuals. Obesity is also a risk factor for underlying cardiovascular problems, which could lead to an increased chance of medical complications post-transplant.

Because of these risk factors, most obese individuals will not be suitable donors. The exact upper limit of BMI is at the discretion of the individual center. Certainly a BMI >35 would be a contraindication for virtually all centers. Many centers will exclude donors with BMI >30, but others will selectively evaluate these donors, and routinely perform a liver biopsy on them to rule out the possibility of liver steatosis [13,14].

Hepatitis B core-antibody-positive donors
The use of donors who are hepatitis B virus (HBV) core-antibody-positive involves consideration of two factors: risk to the donor and potential risk of transmission to the recipient [15]. Donors who are HBV core-positive but surface-antigen-negative have had previous exposure to HBV but do not have active infection. The proportion of potential donors that are core-positive will vary depending on the geographic area. For example, in parts of Asia more than 50% of potential donors may fall into this category. The majority of these donors will have completely normal livers, and studies from centers in Asia have shown that the risk to them is no higher than that to non-HBV core-antibody-positive donors. However, since these donors have had previous HBV infection, a liver biopsy should be performed during the evaluation process to rule out the possibility of hepatic inflammation or fibrosis.

With regard to the recipient, the issues are no different than those for a deceased donor who is core-positive. A recipients who has not been exposed to HBV in the past can potentially acquire primary HBV infection after transplantation from these donors. However, this risk can be minimized or virtually eliminated by the use of appropriate HBV prophylaxis.

Evaluation for thrombophilia
Deep-venous thrombosis (DVT) with subsequent pulmonary embolism represents a serious postoperative complication that can be potentially life-threatening. Several cases of pulmonary embolism have been reported,

with at least one or two cases of mortality due to this complication. Known risk factors for thromboembolic complications include obesity, use of oral hormone therapy, older age, smoking, positive family history, and an identified underlying procoagulation disorder. These risk factors should be addressed during the evaluation process, which should include screening tests to identify a procoagulation disorder. Tests should check for protein C and S deficiency, the presence of antiphospholipid or anticardiolipin antibodies, and factor V Leiden and prothrombin gene mutations.

Surgical evaluation

This part of the evaluation is concerned with determining whether the anatomy of the liver is suitable for donation. A number of tests can be performed here, but essentially one wants to obtain information about the vascular anatomy, the liver volume (both the volume to be removed and the volume to be left behind), and the presence of any abnormalities of the hepatic parenchyma.

Vascular anatomy

Evaluation of the vascular anatomy pre-donation includes imaging of the hepatic artery, portal vein, and hepatic veins. Most centers have abandoned the use of invasive tests such as angiography, and routinely use computed tomography (CT) or magnetic resonance imaging (MRI) with three-dimensional reconstructions as a single test [16,17]. While some vascular variations may preclude donation, most can be handled with vascular-reconstruction techniques. However, preoperative knowledge of these variations is important for planning the operative procedure and performing the operative dissection. Possible vascular variations include a replaced or accessory left (or right) hepatic artery, trifurcation of the main portal vein, and accessory hepatic veins. Depending on which portion of the liver is to be removed, these anatomical variations may either have no impact or significantly complicate surgery.

The biliary anatomy may be difficult to evaluate accurately preoperatively. Some centers routinely perform magnetic resonance cholangiopancre-atography (MRCP) or endoscopic retrograde cholangiopancreatography (ERCP) as part of the evaluation process. The latter is an invasive test, while the former may not provide the degree of accuracy and clarity required to be of value. As a result, many centers choose to perform an intraoperative cholangiogram rather than preoperative biliary imaging. However, ongoing improvements in imaging modalities may soon allow for preoperative noninvasive imaging that is equivalent to the intraoperative cholangiogram with regards to its detail and clarity.

Liver volume

Two important questions need to be answered with regard to liver volume during the evaluation process: (i) Is the volume of the graft to be transplanted of adequate size for the recipient?; and (ii) Is the volume of liver to be left behind in the donor of sufficient size to prevent acute liver failure? While the

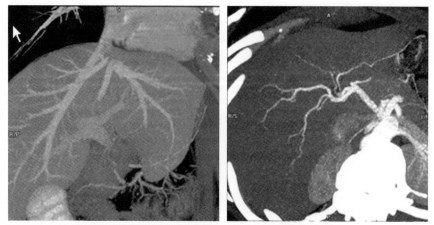

Figure 3.1 Vascular anatomy, including the hepatic veins, portal vein, and hepatic artery, can be determined with a single noninvasive test such as a CT scan with contrast

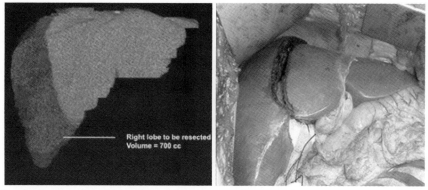

Right lobe to be resected
Volume = 700 cc

Figure 3.2 Determination of the volume of liver to be resected is an important component of the preoperative surgical evaluation and usually correlates well with intraoperative findings

donor's height and weight may provide a crude estimate of liver volume, this will not be very accurate. This is especially true for the left lateral segment, which can be quite variable in size. Again, a CT or MRI scan can provide a good estimate of the liver volume. It is often helpful for the surgeon to work closely with the radiologist in making the planned line of liver transection, in order to provide the most accurate assessment of graft volume (Figures 3.1 and 3.2).

For a pediatric recipient, the main issue is not usually whether the liver volume might be too small, but rather if it might be too large; this can lead to problems with closure of the abdomen in the recipient. Usually the graft-weight-to-recipient-weight (GW/RW) ratio should not exceed 5%. The left lateral segment is used most commonly for these recipients, and removal of this small portion of the liver should not be a concern with regard to adequate residual volume in the donor. For an adult recipient, however, the volume of the graft and residual volume are more critical issues. Most centers currently use the right lobe for adult recipients. Preoperative evaluation should include measurement of the graft liver volume, to ensure that it is not too small for the recipient. Most centers attempt to keep the GW/RW ratio greater than 0.8, or an estimate of graft weight as a percentage of standard liver mass above 40%. Grafts that are smaller than this may be associated with poorer outcome in the recipient, often due to problems such as small-for-size syndrome.

With regard to residual volume in the donor, an important part of the evaluation process is to make sure that the donor is not left with too small a liver volume. Liver failure has been reported post-donation, with at least two donors in the USA having required an urgent liver transplant because of liver failure after donation. The planned resection should not exceed 70% of the total liver volume; that is, the donor should be left with at least 30% of the measured total liver volume.

Liver parenchyma

Evaluation of the liver parenchyma pre-donation is best done with a liver biopsy. The role and utilization of liver biopsy, however, varies from center to center, and remains controversial. Some centers routinely biopsy all potential donors, while others biopsy only on a selective basis [18,19]. The main purpose of the liver biopsy is to assess for the presence and degree of steatosis and rule out any possibility of underlying chronic liver disease. Steatosis may be more common in donors with a history of alcohol use, elevated triglyceride levels, higher BMI, or abnormal appearance on CT imaging. Some centers use these criteria to selectively biopsy the donors. Unfortunately, even with these selection criteria, some cases of steatosis may not be identified pre-donation. Additionally, other parenchymal abnormalities that are occult may be difficult to identify using these criteria, and hence some centers recommend routine biopsy for all potential donors. Liver biopsy represents an invasive test, with a potential risk for complications such as bleeding. However, the risk of complications is generally very low, and may be outweighed by the benefit of identifying a potential donor with significant occult liver disease that would preclude donation. Additional studies are needed to better define the role of liver biopsy.

Liver-biopsy results that would preclude donation include fibrosis, non-alcoholic steatohepatitis (NASH), steatosis >10–20% (for right-lobe liver donors), and histological abnormalities such as inflammatory changes. There are some data to suggest that steatosis identified on a pre-donation biopsy can be reversed with a program of dieting and exercise, and rebiopsy in this situation may show the potential donor to be suitable [20].

Psychosocial evaluation

This part of the evaluation assesses the donor's mental fitness and willingness to donate, ensuring that consent is obtained in a voluntary manner, with the absence of coercion. The formal part of this evaluation should be conducted by a health-care professional such as a psychiatrist, psychologist, social worker, or other mental-health specialist. There are several components to this part of the evaluation, but basically the following issues should be addressed [21–23]:

1. Motivation for donation: The potential donor's reasons for donating need to be determined. This should include a careful assessment to ensure that no coercion or inducement is involved. Some sense of the relationship with the potential recipient should also be obtained.
2. Knowledge of the process: The potential donor must fully understand the donation process, the surgery, the potential complications, and the recovery involved. This is important to obtaining informed consent.
3. Mental health: The mental-health history of the potential donor should be obtained, including underlying psychiatric disorders, history of substance abuse, and overall competence.
4. Psychosocial history: The current psychosocial status of the potential donor should be evaluated, including concurrent stressors, coping strategies, support structures, and stability of living arrangements.
5. Work or school issues: The potential donor's work and financial status, and how the surgery combined with recovery time might impact on this, should be evaluated.

Recipient evaluation

Evaluation of the recipient is similar to that in deceased-donor transplantation and all potential recipients should be listed for deceased-donor liver transplant (DDLT). Particular attention needs to be paid to the degree of underlying portal hypertension, patency of portal and hepatic vasculature, presence of hepatocellular carcinoma (HCC), and cardiac and pulmonary status. Size-matching between the potential donor and the intended recipient is also an essential component of the evaluation.

Pediatric recipients

Introduction

The use of living donors for the acquisition of a liver graft for transplantation into infants and children has become an accepted and highly successful procedure around the world. For a pediatric recipient, the left lateral segment of the donor's liver (about 25% of the total liver) is usually removed. For a larger child, the left lobe is sometimes used. The operative procedure involves isolating the blood vessels supplying the portion of the liver to be removed, transecting the hepatic parenchyma, and then removing the portion to be transplanted. The operative procedure is in part very similar to the procedure for adult/pediatric cadaveric in situ splits. The outflow of the graft is based on the left hepatic vein, while the inflow is based on the left hepatic artery and the left portal vein (Figure 3.3).

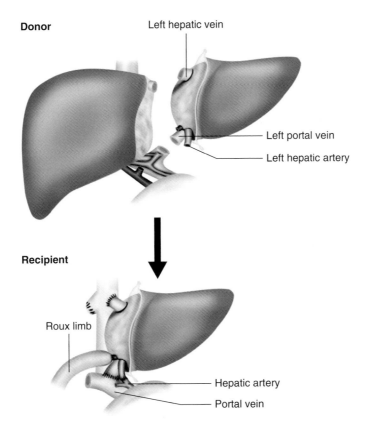

Figure 3.3 Operative procedure for left-lateral-segment LDLT

Donor procedure

The abdomen is opened through a subcostal or midline incision. The falciform ligament and left triangular ligaments are divided up to the anterior aspect of the left hepatic vein. The left lateral segment is lifted up slightly and the gastrohepatic ligament is divided from the hilum posteriorly to the left hepatic vein superiorly. The left hepatic vein is then encircled with an umbilical tape. The bridge of liver tissue overlying the ligamentum teres and connecting the left lateral segment to segment IV is divided; this can usually be done with electrocautery. The left hepatic artery is identified at the base of the ligament of Teres and traced distally to where it enters the liver, and proximally to the segment-IV branch. The left portal vein can be identified and mobilized along its long extrahepatic course, lying slightly superior and posterior to the artery. The falciform ligament is pulled to the left and "feedback vessels" of the portal vein going to segment IV are identified and divided with suture ligation.

The umbilical tape previously passed around the left hepatic vein is brought around the left lateral segment itself, passing in the ligamentum groove, and anteriorly excluding the artery and vein going to the left lateral segment. Pulling on the two ends of the umbilical tape lifts up the portion of liver to be transected, giving a good guide for the plane of transection. This is known as the "hanging technique." The parenchyma of the liver is then transected, staying just to the right of the falciform ligament. As the parenchymal transection is continued, the biliary drainage from segments II and III is encountered, just at the base of the lateral segment, superior to the vascular structures, which are sharply transected. When the recipient team is ready, the graft is removed by dividing the vascular structures. Clamps are placed proximally on the left portal vein and left hepatic artery. The left hepatic vein is most easily taken with an endo-stapling device. The graft is flushed and given to the recipient team. The cut surface of the donor is carefully inspected for any evidence of bleeding or bile leak. Once this is satisfactory, closure is performed.

Recipient operative procedure
A standard caval-preserving hepatectomy is performed while the donor team is procuring the left-lateral-segment graft. Creation of a large, patulous, hepatic venous anastomosis is important to maximize outflow of the graft. This is best performed by isolating the cava between two clamps. A large triangular opening is created on the anterior surface of the cava, usually at the site of the left- and middle-hepatic-vein orifices. Three corner sutures are placed at the angles of the triangle and the corresponding locations on the donor hepatic vein (marking these locations on the donor vein with a marking pen prior to graft implantation is helpful in ensuring proper orientation). The corner sutures are tied and the anastomosis is completed with a running suture technique. A small defect is left to allow for flushing of the graft.

The portal venous anastomosis is completed next. Usually this can be done without the use of a jump graft. Correct orientation of the donor and recipient veins is important to ensuring unobstructed flow. The graft is then flushed to remove preservative solution. After flushing, the defect in the hepatic venous anastomosis is closed and the clamps are removed. Then the hepatic arterial anastomosis is completed. Again, this can usually be done without the use of a "jump" graft. An operating microscope or high-powered Loupes and fine interrupted sutures are helpful in creating this anastomosis. A Roux-en-Y loop is then created for the biliary anastomosis. The loop is brought up through a retrocolic opening and placed adjacent to the bile duct(s), so that a tension-free anastomosis can be performed. It is helpful to perform this anastomosis over a small feeding tube, which can be used as an external stent.

Adult-to-adult LDLT

Introduction
The use of living donors for liver transplant has been of tremendous benefit to pediatric recipients and has resulted in a significant decrease in the waiting-list mortality rate for these patients. However, more than 90%

of patients on the waiting list today are adults; the majority of deaths pretransplant occur in adults. Therefore, to have maximum impact on the waiting list, living donors also need to be utilized for adult recipients. For such recipients, a larger piece of the liver is required.

Adult living-donor transplants: which portion of the liver to use?

As adult-to-adult LDLTs become increasingly popular, debate centers on which portion of the donor's liver constitutes the ideal graft. Almost every portion has been used, including the left lateral segment, left lobe (with or without the caudate lobe), right lobe, and extended right lobe; even dual left-lobe grafts from two separate donors have been used [24]. In deciding which portion is best, donor safety is of primary importance: the risk to the donor must be minimized as much as possible. However, the risk to the donor must be balanced by the benefit to the recipient. A graft with a high likelihood of failure in the recipient is of no benefit to anyone involved in the living-donor process. For example, using smaller portions of the donor's liver might decrease the risk to the donor, but the results could be dismal in the recipient. Conversely, larger portions of the donor's liver might be associated with better results in the recipient, but these should not be removed if it significantly increases the risk to the donor. In the USA, most centers now use the right lobe for adult-to-adult LDLTs. The left lobe is not commonly used, based on results of earlier series reporting a high incidence of small-for-size syndrome and graft loss [25] though more recent series are challenging this. Shimada *et al.* from Kyushu University, Japan, reported 136 cases of adult-to-adult LDLTs using the left lobe and compared the results with 68 cases using the right lobe. The cumulative overall 1-, 3-, and 5-year graft survival rates in recipients of the left lobe were 81.2, 78.8, and 77.2%, respectively—not significantly different from those in recipients of the right lobe. But the overall donor complication rate in right-lobe donors was higher than that in left-lobe donors [26]. Yet reports from centers doing both left-lobe and right-lobe resection did not show any difference in donor mortality or morbidity. Moreover, the general surgical literature on these two types of resection in nontransplant settings has also not shown significant differences in mortality. Still, a right hepatectomy does involve removing a larger mass of the liver and likely entails greater surgical stress for the donor. In the Shimada series, right-lobe donors had higher serum aspartate aminotransferase and bilirubin postoperatively and longer hospital stays. Similar findings were noted in a non-donor model, with patients undergoing hepatic resection for malignancy [27]; recovery of liver function, per laboratory tests, was slower, and morbidity was higher in the right (versus left) hepatectomy patients. Therefore, a left-lobe resection may be safer for liver donors, but again the evidence is inconclusive.

In the transplant literature, results for the recipient have been inferior with the left lobe (versus the right). One main reason is the significantly higher incidence of poor early graft function. This clinical scenario, characterized by persistent hyperbilirubinemia and ascites, is often called small-for-size syndrome. In an earlier report by Ben-Haim *et al.*, of 10 left-lobe recipients, four (40%) had small-for-size syndrome; of 30 right-lobe recipients, only one (3.3%) had a similar problem [25]. Even in the Shimada initial series of 39 left-lobe recipients, 12 (30.8%) had persistent hyperbilirubinemia (defined as serum bilirubin >10 mg/dl on post-transplant day 14). That rate of hyperbilirubinemia was equivalent to the rate in their six right-lobe recipients, yet is higher than the results generally reported in the literature for right-lobe recipients. Nonetheless, these left-lobe grafts recovered, and demonstrated good long-term function.

In deciding whether a left-lobe graft is sufficient for an individual recipient, two factors are likely important: the size of the donor's graft relative to the recipient (expressed as a percentage of the size of the recipient) and the severity of the recipient's liver disease, including the degree of portal hypoperfusion. Graft size can be expressed as a percentage of the calculated ideal liver weight of the recipient (CILW: ideally should be ≥40%) or as a ratio of graft weight to recipient weight (GW/RW: ideally should be ≥0.80%). Thus, because the left lobe of the average donor's liver weighs between 400 and 500 g, such a graft could be used safely for a recipient weighing between 55 and 65 kg. Larger lobes could, of course, be used for larger recipients.

Yet transplants with a GW/RW ratio of <0.8% or with a CILW < 40% have been done with good results, probably because disease severity also impacts on how much liver mass is needed. Recipients with relatively well-compensated cirrhosis and recipients without cirrhosis can likely tolerate a smaller graft size (perhaps GW/RW as low as 0.6%). In this scenario, an average left lobe could then be used for a 70–85 kg recipient with a good chance of success. Measurement of portal pressure and adjustments using modulation techniques like splenic artery ligation or portocaval shunts may help to prevent portal hyperperfusion, which is the likely cause of small-for-size syndrome, and thus can further expand the use of the left lobe. However, for recipients with severe decompensated cirrhosis (Childs C, Model for End-stage Liver Disease (MELD) score >24), a larger graft (such as a right lobe) should be used to provide adequate liver volume and to minimize the risk of small-for-size syndrome.

Inclusion of segment 1 (caudate lobe) with the left-lobe graft, especially if the graft is marginal in size, may be of tremendous benefit. In such cases, the caudate lobe might increase the left-lobe graft by 5–10%. While this is a relatively small increase in size, it may be clinically important. If the caudate lobe is to be preserved with the graft, care must be taken to maintain an adequate blood supply. If the hepatic vein which drains the caudate lobe into the cava is of significant size, it can be preserved and reimplanted in the recipient. Doing so will minimize congestion of the caudate lobe after graft reperfusion [28].

The choice of surgical procedure for adult living-donor transplant varies from center to center, but most prefer the right lobe (Figure 3.4). The recipient operation with LDLTs is not greatly different from that in whole-organ DDLTs. The hepatectomy is performed in a similar fashion, but the recipient cava should be preserved in all cases, because the graft

Donor

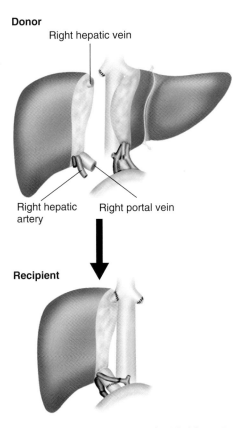

Figure 3.4 Operative procedure for right-lobe LDLT

will generally only have a single hepatic vein for outflow. This hepatic vein is then anastomosed directly to the recipient's preserved vena cava. Outflow can be augmented by including the middle hepatic vein with the graft, or by reconstructing large segment-V or VIII tributaries to the middle hepatic vein using a vascular conduit. Inflow to the graft can be achieved by reconnecting the corresponding hepatic arterial and portal venous branches. Finally, biliary reconstruction is performed either by a duct-to-duct technique or with a hepaticojejunostomy.

Donor operative procedure: right lobe

A bilateral subcostal incision is usually used. The falciform ligament is divided and then continued posteriorly until the anterior wall of the right hepatic vein is visualized. The right lobe of the liver is completely mobilized by division of the right triangular ligament and freeing of the bare area from the underlying retroperitoneum. The right lobe is mobilized from the retrohepatic cava itself by dividing the short hepatic veins that drain into the cava. Any branches 5 mm or larger should be preserved for later reimplantation in the recipient. The right hepatic vein is encircled after mobilization of the lobe. Attention is then turned toward the hilar dissection. A cholecystectomy is performed. The right-hilar plate is taken down and the junction of the right and left hepatic ducts is defined. The right hepatic artery is identified close to where it enters into the liver and is then traced proximally to the point where it usually passes behind the common bile duct (CBD). It should not normally be dissected much proximal to this point, so as not to risk causing vascular injury to the CBD. The right portal vein is then identified. The junction with the left portal vein is clearly defined, so as to not compromise the latter when the right portal vein is eventually divided. The right hepatic artery and right portal vein are retracted inferiorly and the right hepatic duct is encircled. An intraoperative cholangiogram is then performed to delineate the biliary anatomy.

Intraoperative ultrasound is performed to outline the course of the middle hepatic vein. This is correlated with the preoperative imaging study. We prefer to perform the parenchymal transection just to the right of the middle hepatic vein, leaving that structure with the donor. Others have described doing the parenchymal transection to the left of the middle hepatic vein, leaving it with the right-lobe graft. The ultrasound is also useful in helping identify large venous tributaries draining segment V and/or VIII into the middle hepatic vein. The location of these can be marked on the surface of the liver, which is useful during the parenchymal transection. If large (>4 mm), they may need to be reconstructed in the recipient.

Parenchymal transection is then performed, and during this it is helpful to keep the central venous pressure in the donor low, so as to minimize bleeding. When any large tributaries (>4 mm) draining into the middle hepatic vein are encountered, they can be divided and tagged for later reimplantation in the recipient. Once the parenchymal transection is completed, the right hepatic duct is divided at the determined site, based on the cholangiogram. The corresponding biliary stump on the left side is closed, taking care not to narrow the common hepatic duct.

We prefer to wait at this point until the recipient team is ready to receive the liver. This also allows for close inspection of the two pieces of the liver, to ensure that they are both adequately perfused. When the recipient team is ready, the vascular structures of the right graft are divided. The right hepatic artery is taken first, with a vascular clamp. The right portal vein is divided next, either using a vascular clamp or a linear stapling device for proximal control. Regardless of how control is achieved, it is important that the stump of the right portal vein is closed in an anterior-to-posterior fashion, rather than a side-to-side manner. This ensures that there is no narrowing at the junction between the left and main portal veins.

The right hepatic vein is easiest to divide using a laparoscopic stapling device. The right lobe is removed and given to the recipient team. The cut surface of the left lobe is carefully inspected for any evidence of bile leak or bleeding. The falciform ligament is reattached using a running suture, to prevent torsion of the remaining left lobe. We prefer to leave a drain in place, but many centers do not.

Donor operative procedure: left lobe

The abdomen is opened through a subcostal incision. The falciform ligament and left triangular ligaments are divided up to the anterior aspect of the left hepatic vein. The left lateral segment is lifted slightly and the gastrohepatic ligament is divided from the hilum posteriorly to the left hepatic vein superiorly. The Caudate lobe is dissected off of the inferior vena cava by dividing the minor hepatic veins. A large caudate hepatic vein near the midline of the inferior vena cava is present in 70% cases and should be preserved with the graft for subsequent implantation. Cholecystectomy and intraoperative cholangiogram are then performed to delineate the biliary anatomy. Attention is next turned toward the hilar dissection. The left hepatic artery is dissected proximally up to bifurcation, preserving the segment-IV artery. The left portal vein is identified medial and posterior to left hepatic artery and dissected circumferentially.

The umbilical tape is then passed behind the caudate lobe through the groove between the right and middle hepatic veins, to facilitate parenchymal transaction. Intraoperative ultrasound is performed to outline the course of the middle hepatic vein. The parenchyma of the liver is transected, staying just to the right of middle hepatic vein. As the parenchymal transection is continued to the hilar plate, the biliary system is encountered and the left hepatic duct is sharply transected. Careful search is made for any caudate hepatic duct, and it is incorporated into the left hepatic duct, or implanted separately if it is large.

When the recipient team is ready, the graft is removed by dividing the vascular structures. Clamps are placed proximally on the left portal vein and left hepatic artery. The common trunk of the left and middle hepatic veins is taken with an endo-stapling device. The graft is flushed and given to the recipient team. The cut surface of the donor is carefully inspected for any evidence of bleeding or bile leak. Once this is satisfactory, closure is performed.

Recipient operative procedure (right lobe)

The graft is flushed with preservative solution and weighed. If there are any segment-V or VIII veins that will need to be reimplanted (based on size being ≥5 mm) then a conduit of some form can be utilized. Options include using a cryopreserved vein, the recipient's saphenous or superficial femoral vein, a segment of vein from the resected liver (such as the left portal vein), or a vessel from a deceased donor.

A standard inferior-vena-cava-sparing hepatectomy is done in the recipient; the liver is mobilized off the underlying cava and all short hepatic veins are divided. The orifices of the three hepatic veins are stapled shut and the liver is removed completely. The donor right hepatic vein is anastomosed to a venotomy made on the anterior wall of the cava. It is important to have a nice patulous anastomosis to maximize outflow. The donor right portal vein is anastomosed to the recipient main portal vein. Any middle-hepatic-vein tributaries that have been reconstructed can be reimplanted directly to the cava, or the orifies of the recipient middle/left hepatic vein.

The donor right hepatic artery is anastomosed to the recipient right hepatic artery using fine interrupted sutures. Finally, the bile ducts are reconstructed. If the recipient bile duct reaches the donor bile duct without tension, a duct-to-duct anastomosis can be done. Even when there are two ducts in the donor graft, as long as the recipient ducts have been divided high in the hilum, a duct-to-duct anastomosis is possible to the native right and left hepatic ducts. It is helpful to perform this anastomosis over an internal stent. Alternatively, a Roux-en-Y loop can be used if it is not possible to use the recipient's own ducts. Using an external biliary stent is helpful when performing this anastomosis, and allows for easy imaging afterward.

Donor outcome

Donor mortality
The greatest concern with LDLT, in fact with any living-donor procedure, is the risk of death to the donor. Unfortunately, there is some risk of mortality associated with any surgical procedure, but the magnitude of risk associated with this procedure has been difficult to determine. As of February 28, 2010, 2753 adult and 1283 pediatric LDLTs had been performed in the USA and reported to UNOS (United Network for Organ Sharing) [1], among which were seven donor deaths (0.2%) [10]. Of these seven deaths, three were early in the postoperative period and directly related to the surgery [29] and the remainder were late and likely not related to the donation surgery. The number of deaths worldwide, however, is more difficult to know, as there is no mandatory reporting. By some reports, there have been 19 deaths worldwide [30]. Most centers will quote a 0.5% risk of mortality associated with this procedure, though the quoted rate may vary from 0.1 to 1.0% at different centers. Based on the deaths described in world literature, the overall mortality rate is of the order of 0.2–0.5%. The estimated mortality for donation for a pediatric recipient is lower than that for donation for an adult recipient, likely as a result of the magnitude of liver resection involved. Similarly, the risk associated with left-lobe donation may be lower than that with right-lobe donation.

Donor morbidity
The reported incidence of complications in the donor varies in the literature from 9 to 67%, but is likely in the 30% range [31–36]. A number of different complications have been reported in donors. The vast majority tend to occur in the early postoperative period (usually within 1 month post-donation). The modified Clavien classification is commonly used to describe, report, and compare donor morbidity: Grade I—a complication that is not life-threatening, does not result in residual disability, and does not require a therapeutic invasive intervention; Grade II—a complication that is potentially life-threatening and that requires the use of drug therapy or foreign blood units; Grade III—a complication that is potentially life-threatening and that requires a therapeutic invasive intervention; Grade IV—a complication with residual or lasting disability or which leads to

death [31]. The Adult Living Donor Liver Transplantation Cohort Study (A2ALL), funded by the National Institutes of Health, with nine liver-transplant centers, reported a donor complication rate of 38%; 21% of donors had one complication and 17% had two or more. Complications were graded using the modified Clavien system described above: 27% had grade-I (minor), 26% had grade-II (potentially life-threatening), 2% had grade-III (life-threatening), and 0.8% had grade-IV (leading to death) complications. Common complications included biliary leaks beyond post-operative day 7 (9%), bacterial infections (12%), incisional hernia (6%), pleural effusion requiring intervention (5%), neuropraxia (4%), reexploration (3%), wound infections (3%), and intraabdominal abscess (2%). Two donors developed portal-vein thrombosis and one had inferior vena-caval thrombosis; 13% of donors required hospital readmission and 4% required two to five readmissions [36].

Biliary problems are the most common major complication after donor surgery. Bile leaks and strictures have been reported in roughly 10 and 3% of donors, respectively. Bile may leak from the cut surface of the liver or from the site where the bile duct is divided. That site may later become strictured. Generally, bile leaks resolve spontaneously with simple drainage. Strictures and sometimes bile leaks may require an endoscopic procedure and stenting. If these measures fail, a reoperation may be required. Intra-abdominal infections developing in donors are usually related to a biliary problem [37].

Hemorrhage is another major complication. It can be intraoperative or postoperative. Intraoperative blood loss is usually in the range of 250–750 cc for uncomplicated cases and depends on the transection surface, the anatomy of the vessels, and most importantly the experience and skill of the surgeons. Blood loss can be reduced by keeping the central venous pressure low. The risk of postoperative blood loss requiring nonautologous blood and the need for reoperation is usually less than 5% [31,32,35].

Liver-function recovery and liver regeneration

Liver enzymes usually peak early in the first 48–72 hours after surgery, with serum bilirubin generally peaking 1 or 2 days after. Synthetic liver-function tests are usually fairly normal by 1 week postoperatively. Volume studies generally show that the liver remnant achieves 80–90% of its ideal liver volume by 3 months post-surgery [38].

Recipient outcome

Living-donor recipients have been noted to have a higher incidence of surgical complications post-transplant compared with whole-liver recipients. Early data suggested that outcomes (graft survival) might be inferior to those in whole-liver transplants, especially if the patients were matched for severity of liver disease [39]. Partial grafts have smaller vessels, more complicated biliary reconstructions, and a cut surface, all of which make for a technically more challenging procedure and a higher incidence of surgical complications. Maluf *et al.* and Fan *et al.* reported that despite smaller graft size and higher technical complexity, the graft and patient survival rates of patients with right-liver LDLT are not different from those of patients receiving whole-graft DDLT [40,41]. The only difference is a higher incidence of biliary complications in the LDLT patients (25.8 versus 7.1%) [40].

Most centers have reported a 15–46% incidence of biliary complications, including early bile leaks, after transplant, and a 15–20% incidence of late biliary strictures. These figures are significantly higher than are generally reported for whole-liver recipients (9–15%) [40]. The possible factors associated with an increased risk of postoperative biliary complications include having multiple bile ducts to reconstruct and an inadequate arterial perfusion in patients with a high preoperative MELD score [42,43].

With advances in microsurgical techniques, the incidence of vascular complications such as hepatic artery thrombosis has decreased and is now not significantly different from that in deceased-liver transplants [44–47].

Certain subgroups of recipients may do worse after living-donor transplants. Critically ill adult recipients with advanced liver failure, high MELD scores, and numerous secondary complications have generally been reported to have worse outcomes with this procedure. Such recipients have minimal functional reserve and are probably ill equipped to manage the lower hepatocyte mass and the higher complication rate associated with partial transplants. However, in parts of the world where DDLTs are uncommon, living donors have been used for critically ill patients, with good results [40].

Small-for-size syndrome

Small-for-size syndrome has emerged as an interesting and significant problem that is fairly unique to partial-liver transplants. Small-for-size syndrome and injury related to the use of small-for-size grafts were initially reported in 1996 by Emond *et al.* [48]. Although there is no uniform consensus on the definition of small-for-size syndrome, a diagnosis of small-for-size-graft syndrome is generally based on persistent hyperbilirubinemia and massive ascites during the post-transplant subacute phase, without evidence of any other cause [49–51]. The incidence is reportedly close to 10%, although this cannot be known exactly as the definition for this condition is not agreed upon. Multiple risk factors have been identified, including the size of the graft, the type of graft, the degree of portal hypertension, and the spleen size. Of these, the degree of portal hypertension (and portal perfusion) is likely most important [52]. The pathophysiology of the condition is believed to be related to damage to hepatocytes and vasculature secondary to portal shear stress. Portal hyperperfusion leads to poor hepatic arterial inflow due to the arterial buffer response, which ultimately leads to hepatic necrosis and poor hepatic regeneration [53].

In the absence of any intervention, small-for-size syndrome is associated with a significant mortality early post-transplant, with many patients succumbing to complications associated with poor graft function, such as infections and multiorgan failure. With increased understanding of the

Table 3.1 Mechanisms of small-for-size syndrome and associated strategies by which to address them.

	Mechanism of SFSS	Strategies
Strategies to prevent SFSS	Suboptimal Graft Quality	Younger Donor, Non fatty Liver, Decrease Ischemia time
	Insufficient Graft Volume	Adequate Graft Volume (CILW: ideally should be $\geq$ 40%), (GW/RW: ideally should be $\geq$ 0.80%)
Strategies to Rescue	Increased portal Flow	Porto-Systemic Shunt, Splenectomy. Splenic Artery Ligation
	Impaired Venous Outflow	Inclusion of MHV in graft, Wide Venous anastomosis, Reconstruction of Segmental drainage

concept of small-for-size, strategies to prevent small-for-size syndrome and to rescue small-for-size grafts are being developed (Table 3.1).

Conclusion

LDLT has evolved as an alternative to DDLT for patients with end-stage liver disease. While there is no obvious benefit for donors, there are advantages to recipients of living-donor transplants. In countries without DDLT, the survival benefit associated with LDLT is obvious. Even in areas with DDLT, the potential risk of mortality associated with waiting for a deceased donor is avoided. Additionally, patients can be transplanted before they develop far-advanced liver disease associated with marked overall decompensation. These factors have become especially helpful for patients who are disadvantaged by deceased-organ allocation schemes. While the advantages of live-donor transplants to potential recipients are obvious, this must be carefully balanced against the risk of mortality and morbidity for the donor. Short-term and long-term results in the donor must be carefully tracked and the technique must be refined to try to minimize this risk as much as possible.

References

1 http://optn.transplant.hrsa.gov/.
2 Smith B. Segmental liver transplantation from a living donor. *J Pediatr Surg* 1969;4:126–132.
3 Raia S, Nery JR, Mies S. Liver transplantation from live donors. *Lancet* 1989;2:497.
4 Strong RW, Lynch SV, Ong TH, Matsunami H, Koido Y, Balderson GA. Successful liver transplantation from a living donor to her son. *N Engl J Med* 1990;322:1505–1507.

5 Broelsch CE, Emond JC, Whitington PF, Thistlethwaite JR, Baker AL, Lichtor JL. Application of reduced-size liver transplants as split grafts, auxiliary orthotopic grafts, and living related segmental transplants. *Ann Surg* 1990;212(3):368–375.

6 Hashikura Y, Makuuchi M, Kawasaki S, Matsunami H, Ikegami T, Nakazawa Y, Kiyosawa K, Ichida T. Successful living-related partial liver transplantation to an adult patient. *Lancet* 1994;343:1233–1234.

7 Yamaoka Y, Washida M, Honda K, Tanaka K, Mori K, Shimahara Y, Okamoto S, Ueda M, Hayashi M, Tanaka A. Liver transplantation using a right lobe graft from a living related donor. *Transplantation* 1994;57:1127–1130.

8 Lo CM, Fan ST, Liu CL, Lo RJ, Lau GK, Wei WI, Li JH, Ng IO, Wong J. Extending the limit on the size of adult recipient in living donor liver transplantation using extended right lobe graft. *Transplantation* 1997;63:1524–1528.

9 Wachs ME, Bak TE, Karrer FM, Everson GT, Shrestha R, Trouillot TE, Mandell MS, Steinberg TG, Kam I. Adult living donor liver transplantation using a right hepatic lobe. *Transplantation* 1998;66(10):1313–1316.

10 Surman OS. The ethics of partial liver donation. *New Engl J Med* 2002;346(14):1038.

11 Rudow DL, Brown RS Jr., Evaluation of living liver donors. *Prog Transplant* 2003;13(2):110–116.

12 Rinella ME, Alonso E, Rao S, Whitington P, Fryer J, Abecassis M, Superina R, Flamm SL, Blei AT. Body mass index as a predictor of hepatic steatosis in living liver donors. *Liver Transpl* 2001;7(5):409–414.

13 Trotter JF, Wachs M, Trouillot T, Steinberg T, Bak T, Everson GT, Kam I. Evaluation of 100 patients for living donor liver transplantation. *Liver Transpl* 2000;6(3):290–295.

14 Trotter JF. Selection of donors and recipients for living donor liver transplantation. *Liver Transpl* 2000;6(6 Suppl 2):S52–S58.

15 Chen YS, Cheng YF, De Villa VH, Wang CC, Lin CC, Huang TL, Jawan B, Chen CL. Evaluation of living liver donors. *Transplantation* 2003;75 (3 Suppl):S16–S19.

16 Alonso-Torres A, Fernandez-Cuadrado J, Pinilla I, Parron M, de Vicente E, Lopez-Santamaria M. Multidetector CT in the evaluation of potential living donors for liver transplantation. *Radiographics* 2005;25(4):1017–1030.

17 Valentin-Gamazo C, Malago M, Karliova M, Lutz JT, Frilling A, Nadalin S, Testa G, Ruehm SG, Erim Y, Paul A, Lang H, Gerken G, Broelsch CE. Experience after the evaluation of 700 potential donors for living donor liver transplantation in a single center. *Liver Transpl* 2004;10(9):1087–1096.

18 Nadalin S, Malago M, Valentin-Gamazo C, Testa G, Baba HA, Liu C, Fruhauf NR, Schaffer R, Gerken G, Frilling A, Broelsch CE. Preoperative donor liver biopsy for adult living donor liver transplantation: risks and benefits. *Liver Transpl* 2005;11(8):980–986.

19 Iwasaki M, Takada Y, Hayashi M, Minamiguchi S, Haga H, Maetani Y, Fujii K, Kiuchi T, Tanaka K Noninvasive evaluation of graft steatosis in living donor liver transplantation. *Transplantation* 2004;78(10):1501–1505.

20 Nakamuta M, Morizono S, Soejima Y, Yoshizumi T, Aishima S, Takasugi S, Yoshimitsu K, Enjoji M, Kotoh K, Taketomi A, Uchiyama H, Shimada M, Nawata H, Maehara Y. Short-term intensive treatment for donors with hepatic steatosis in living-donor liver transplantation. *Transplantation* 2005;80(5):608–612.

21 Jacobs C, Johnson E, Anderson K, Gillingham K, Matas A. Kidney transplants from living donors: how donation affects family dynamics. *Adv Ren Replace Ther* 1998;5(2):89–97.

22 Pradel FG, Mullins CD, Bartlett ST. Exploring donors' and recipients' attitudes about living donor kidney transplantation. *Prog Transplant* 2003;13(3):203–210.

23 Schover LR, Streem SB, Boparai N, Duriak K, Novick AC. The psychosocial impact of donating a kidney: long-term follow-up from a urology based center. *J Urol* 1997;157(5):1596–1601.

24 Lee SG, Park KM, Hwang S, Lee YJ, Kim KH, Ahn CS, Choi DL, Joo SH, Jeon JY, Chu CW, Moon DB, Min PC, Koh KS, Han SH, Park SH, Choi GT, Hwang KS, Lee EJ, Chung YH, Lee YS, Lee HJ, Kim MH, Lee SK, Suh DJ, Kim JJ, Sung KB. Adult-to-adult living donor liver transplantation at the Asan Medical Center, Korea. *Asian J Surg* 2002;25(4):277–284.

25 Ben-Haim M, Emre S, Fishbein T, Sheiner P, Bodian C, Kim-Schluger L, Schwartz M, Miller C. Critical graft size in adult-to-adult living donor liver transplantation: impact of the recipient's disease. *Liver Transplantation* 2001;7(11):948–953.

26 Taketomi A, Kayashima H, Soejima Y, Yoshizumi T, Uchiyama H, Ikegami T, Yamashita Y, Harada N, Shimada M, Maehara Y. Donor risk in adult-to-adult living donor liver transplantation: impact of left lobe graft. *Transplantation* 2009;87(3):445–450.

27 Kanoh K, Nomoto K, Shimura T, Shimada M, Sugimachi K, Kuwano H. A comparison of right-lobe and left-lobe graft for living-donor liver transplantation. *Hepatogastroenterology* 2002;49(43):222–224.

28 Ikegami T, Nishizaki T, Yanaga K, Shimada M, Kakizoe S, Nomoto K, Hiroshige S, Sugimachi K. Changes in the caudate lobe that is transplanted with extended left lobe liver graft from living donors. *Surgery* 2001;129(1):86–90.

29 Middleton PF, Duffield M, Lynch SV, Padbury RT, House T, Stanton P, Verran D, Maddern G. Living donor liver transplantation—adult donor outcomes: a systematic review. *Liver Transpl* 2006;12(1):24–30.

30 Trotter JF, Adam R, Lo CM, Kenison J. Documented deaths of hepatic lobe donors for living donor liver transplantation. *Liver Transpl* 2006;12(10): 1485–1488.

31 Salvalaggio PR, Baker TB, Koffron AJ, *et al.* Comparative analysis of live liver donation risk using a comprehensive grading system for severity. *Transplantation* 2004;77:1765.

32 Brown RS Jr., Russo MW, Lai M, *et al.* A survey of liver transplantation from living adult donors in the United States. *N Engl J Med* 2003;348(9):818.

33 Lo CM. Complications and long-term outcome of living liver donors: a survey of 1508 cases in five Asian centers. *Transplantation* 2003;75(Suppl):S12.

34 Umeshita K, Fujiwara K, Kiyosawa K, *et al.* Operative morbidity of living liver donors in Japan. *Lancet* 2003;362(9385):687.

35 Broering DC, Wilms C, Bok P, Fischer L, Mueller L, Hillert C, Lenk C, Kim JS, Sterneck M, Schulz KH, Krupski G, Nierhaus A, Ameis D, Burdelski M, Rogiers X. Evolution of donor morbidity in living related liver transplantation: a single-center analysis of 165 cases. *Ann Surg* 2004;240(6):1013–1024, disc. 1024–1026.

36 Ghobrial RM, Freise CE, Trotter JF, Tong L, Ojo AO, Fair JH, Fisher RA, Emond JC, Koffron AJ, Pruett TL, Olthoff KM; A2ALL Study Group. Donor

morbidity after living donation for liver transplantation. *Gastroenterology* 2008;135(2):468–476.

37 Yuan Y, Gotoh M. Biliary complications in living liver donors. *Surg Today* 2010;40(5):411–417.

38 Humar A, Kosari K, Sielaff TD, Glessing B, Gomes M, Dietz C, Rosen G, Lake J, Payne WD. Liver regeneration after adult living donor and deceased donor split-liver transplants. *Liver Transpl* 2004;10(3):374–378.

39 Thuluvath PJ, Yoo HY. Graft and patient survival after adult live donor liver transplantation compared to a matched cohort who received a deceased donor transplantation. *Liver Transpl* 2004;10(10):1263–1268.

40 Liu CL, Fan ST, Lo CM, Wei WI, Chan SC, Yong BH, Wong J. Operative outcomes of adult-to-adult right lobe live donor liver transplantation: a comparative study with cadaveric whole-graft liver transplantation in a single center. *Ann Surg* 2006;243:404–410.

41 Maluf DG, Stravitz RT, Cotterell AH, Posner MP, Nakatsuka M, Sterling RK, Luketic VA, Shiffman ML, Ham JM, Marcos A, Behnke MK, Fisher RA. Adult living donor versus deceased donor liver transplantation: a 6-year single center experience. *Am J Transplant* 2005;5:149–156.

42 Liu CL, Lo CM, Chan SC, Fan ST. Safety of duct-to-duct biliary reconstruction in right-lobe live-donor liver transplantation without biliary drainage. *Transplantation* 2004;77(5):726–732.

43 Gondolesi GE, Varotti G, Florman SS, Muñoz L, Fishbein TM, Emre SH, Schwartz ME, Miller C. Biliary complications in 96 consecutive right lobe living donor transplant recipients. *Transplantation* 2004;77(12): 1842–1848.

44 Stange BJ, Glanemann M, Nuessler NC, Settmacher U, Steinmüller T, Neuhaus P. Hepatic artery thrombosis after adult liver transplantation. *Liver Transpl* 2003;9(6):612–620.

45 Bekker J, Ploem S, de Jong KP. Early hepatic artery thrombosis after liver transplantation: a systematic review of the incidence, outcome and risk factors. *Am J Transplant* 2009;9(4):746–757.

46 Miller CM, Gondolesi GE, Florman S, Matsumoto C, Muñoz L, Yoshizumi T, Artis T, Fishbein TM, Sheiner PA, Kim-Schluger L, Schiano T, Shneider BL, Emre S, Schwartz ME. One hundred nine living donor liver transplants in adults and children: a single-center experience. *Ann Surg* 2001;234(3): 301–311.

47 Marcos A, Killackey M, Orloff MS, Mieles L, Bozorgzadeh A, Tan HP. Hepatic arterial reconstruction in 95 adult right lobe living donor liver transplants: evolution of anastomotic technique. *Liver Transpl* 2003;9(6):570–574.

48 Emond JC, Renz JF, Ferrell LD, Rosenthal P, Lim RC, Roberts JP, *et al.* Functional analysis of grafts from living donors. Implications for the treatment of older recipients. *Ann Surg* 1996;224:544–552.

49 Kiuchi T, Tanaka K, Ito T, Oike F, Ogura Y, Fujimoto Y, *et al.* Small-for-size graft in living donor liver transplantation: how far should we go? *Liver Transpl* 2003;9:S29–S35.

50 Imura S, Shimada M, Ikegami T, Morine Y, Kanemura H. Strategies for improving the outcomes in the use of small-for-size grafts in living donor liver transplantation. *J Hepatobiliary Pancreat Surg* 2008;15:102–110.

51 Dahm F, Georgiev P, Clavien PA. Small-for-size syndrome after partial liver transplantation: definition, mechanisms of disease and clinical implications. *Am J Transplant* 2005;5:2605–2610.

52 Troisi R, Ricciardi S, Smeets P, Petrovic M, Van Maele G, Colle I, *et al.* Effects of hemi-portocaval shunts for inflow modulation on the outcome of small-for-size grafts in living donor liver transplantation. *Am J Transplant* 2005;5:1397–1404.

53 Demetris AJ, Kelly DM, Eghtesad B, Fontes P, Wallis Marsh J, *et al.* Pathophysiologic observations and histopathologic recognition of the portal hyperperfusion or small-for-size syndrome. *Am J Surg Pathol* 2006;30:986–993.

4 Antibody-incompatible Transplantation

Nizam Mamode

Guy's and St Thomas' Hospital, Great Ormond Street Hospital, UK

Introduction

Antibody incompatibility has been a central issue in renal transplantation from the beginning; over 50 years ago, Hume and colleagues at the Brigham Hospital described early attempts to transplant kidneys into the thigh [1]. In reporting their experience, they described the transplantation of a kidney from a blood-group-B donor into a 28-year-old, blood-group-O female recipient. After initial function, urine output decreased, and the organ was removed after 7 days. Histology showed infarction of the kidney. This would appear to be the first recorded case of blood-group-incompatible transplantation, and it suggests the development of hyperacute rejection. Subsequently, seminal work in the 1960s by Terasaki and colleagues determined the importance of human leukocyte antigen (HLA) antibodies in transplantation [2] and the need for a negative crossmatch prior to implantation. With the recognition that allografts were doomed to fail in the presence of significant circulating antibody in the recipient against donor antigens, antibody-incompatible transplantation (AIT) was rarely performed until the 1980s, when several groups began to attempt antibody removal in order to avoid hyperacute rejection [3,4]. By the last decade of the 20th century, a mismatch between organ supply and demand generated more interest in AIT; results improved and larger series were reported [5,6], so that currently many large-volume transplant centers have an antibody-incompatible program.

There is little doubt that antibody incompatibility is a major problem in the 21st century. Although estimates vary, some 6000 patients with an antibody-incompatible donor remain on the deceased-donor list in the USA [7]; between 15 and 30% of those presenting for transplantation have an antibody-incompatible donor [8–10], and many will remain on the waiting list, since incompatibility against their living donor may also indicate difficulty in obtaining a deceased-donor organ, particularly with significant HLA sensitization.

Abdominal Organ Transplantation: State of the Art, First Edition.
Edited by Nizam Mamode and Raja Kandaswamy.
© 2013 Blackwell Publishing Ltd. Published 2013 by Blackwell Publishing Ltd.

What has also become clear is that outcomes after HLA-incompatible transplantation (HLAi) are significantly different from those following blood-group-incompatible transplantation (ABOi); the latter is often more easily performed, and has excellent graft and patient survival rates. For this reason, this chapter considers each of these categories separately, and in addition looks at alternatives to AIT, such as paired-exchange schemes. The chapter ends with a summary of how we might approach transplantation in an individual patient with antibody incompatibility.

Blood-group-incompatible transplantation

Hemagglutinins

Blood-group antigens were initially described early in the 20th century by the Austrian biologist Karl Landsteiner, who characterized hemagglutinins present on red blood cells and the corresponding presence (or lack) of antibody in the serum, as shown in Table 4.1. Thus, individuals with antibody against a particular agglutinin would be expected to react to blood containing that antigen. However, for the purposes of transplantation, the issue is more complex. First, although these antigens are expressed on red cells, they are not expressed equally on all other tissues, as shown in Table 4.2. It is clear that ABOi will potentially be more difficult in kidney or pancreas recipients—since there is a high level of expression in these organs—but easier in heart and liver recipients. Indeed, cardiac ABOi has been well-established for some years. Second, as described later, hemagglutinin antibody titers can vary, and this may affect the ease of transplantation.

The hemagglutinin molecule is derived by the action of glycosyl transferase on a core chain, substance H, which is a glycoprotein [11]. Group-A individuals (who are subdivided into A_1 and A_2) have N-acetylgalactosamine added to the core chain, while group-B have D-galactose added. No terminal residues are added to the core chain in group-O individuals. There are four types of H core chain, but it is noteworthy that although in group A_1 glycosyltransferase acts on all four, in group B and in group A_2 only types 1 and 2 are used. Furthermore, as shown in Table 4.2, core-chain expression varies in different tissues, and in the kidney is mainly type 4, with low expression of types 1 and 2. For this reason, groups A_2 and B are said to be less antigenic than A_1.

Table 4.1 Blood-group antigens and antibodies.

Phenotype	Genotype	Antigens	Antibodies	Frequency in UK
O	OO	None	Anti-A & anti-B	44%
A	AA or AO	A	Anti-B	45%
B	BB or BO	B	Anti-A	8%
AB	AB	A & B	None	3%

Table 4.2 Hemagglutinin core-chain H distribution in various human tissues. After [11].

	H chain			
	1	2	3	4
RBC	+	+++	++	+
Plasma	+++	+	+	−
Vascular tissue	++	+	++	−
Liver	++	−	−	−
Pancreas	+++	+	+	
Kidney	+	+	+	+++
Ureter epithelial cells	+		−	++
Stomach	+++		−	−
Small intestine epithelial cells	+++	+	+	−
Large intestine epithelial cells	+++	+	−	−

Reproduced from [11] Rydberg 2001 with permission from John Wiley & Sons Ltd.

Early experience of ABOi therefore focused on A_2 donors, with a report of 50 such cases resulting in a 2-year graft-survival rate of 94%, using OKT3 or antithymocyte globulin (ATG) but without plasma exchange or splenectomy [12].

Hemagglutinin antibody

Isohemagglutinin antibody titers are conventionally expressed in dilutions (negative, neat, 1 in 2, etc.). A variety of methods exist to determine the presence of antibodies; a gel and tube hemagglutination are the most common. There is, however, the potential for considerable variation in technique in this method, both between and within laboratories. A recent study from three of the most experienced centers undertaking ABOi in Europe showed a *median* variation of three titer steps when the same samples were sent to all three laboratories [13]. This was reduced to a median difference of one titer step when the gel technique using Diamed cards was adopted at all institutions, and indeed this is the technique used at Guy's Hospital. Direct and indirect agglutination is performed, on the basis that this allows assessment of both immunoglobulin G and M (IgG and IgM) antibodies, but currently the exact significance of IgM antibodies is unknown. Clearly, inaccurate assessment of titer levels could have dire clinical consequences. It is uncertain whether the use of donor red cells or blood from volunteers with the same blood group is important.

Newer techniques, such as the use of flow cytometry, have been advocated in an attempt to standardize results, but these have not yet been widely adopted [14]. Nevertheless, it is vital for centers to ensure that they are obtaining consistent and reliable results when assessing hemagglutinin titers.

Principles of ABOi transplantation

There are two fundamental principles of ABOi transplantation: first to remove the hemagglutinin antibody, and second to prevent it recurring. The first is relatively straightforward, while the second is a matter of some debate. Each will be discussed in turn.

Antibody removal prior to transplantation

There are currently essentially three methods of removing antibody prior to transplantation: plasma exchange (or variations on this technique), nonspecific immunoabsorption, and antigen-specific immunoabsorption.

Plasma exchange, or plasmapheresis, involves the separation of the patient's blood into a cellular component and plasma, after which the plasma is replaced with albumin or fresh-frozen plasma (FFP) and the components are recombined and returned to the body. This results in the removal of plasma proteins, including hemagglutinins, but as a consequence beneficial proteins, such as clotting factors, may be lost. After several sessions of plasma exchange, it is common for clotting to be significantly deranged, with a prolonged INR and low plasma fibrinogen. Clearly the risks of surgery in this situation are dramatically increased. A refinement of plasma exchange, double-filtration plasmapheresis (DFPP—Figure 4.1), involves two separations and the use of a microfilter that removes high-molecular weight proteins, thus allowing preservation of a significant component of plasma proteins. Hypoalbuminemia and coagulopathy are less likely, but will still occur in prolonged courses of therapy. Larger plasma volumes can be processed due to the decreased fluid loss. Correction of coagulopathy prior to surgery may be done with FFP (which should be either group AB or the donor's blood group, to avoid introduction of hemagglutinins), cryoprecipitate, or fibrinogen, according to local protocol. At Guy's Hospital, fibrinogen is given if the plasma level is below 1 g/l on the day of surgery.

Immunoabsorption requires the use of a plasma separator, followed by passage of plasma through an absorbent column. Nonspecific immunoabsorption has previously been carried out using protein-A columns, but currently the most frequently used column is TheraSorb. The former is derived from staphylococcal proteins which bind human immunoglobulin, while the latter uses sheep-derived polyclonal antihuman antibody bound to a sepharose matrix [15]. The TheraSorb system allows reduction in both IgG (approximately 70% per treatment) and IgM (50% per treatment) antibody, and will remove both HLA antibody and hemagglutinins [16]. It appears to be more effective at removing antibody across all IgG subclasses when compared with the protein-A column. [17] Due to the lack of complete specificity, albumin is reduced by around 20%. The significant advantage of the TheraSorb column is the fact that it may be reused for up to 10 treatments, making it currently relatively cost-effective, as well the

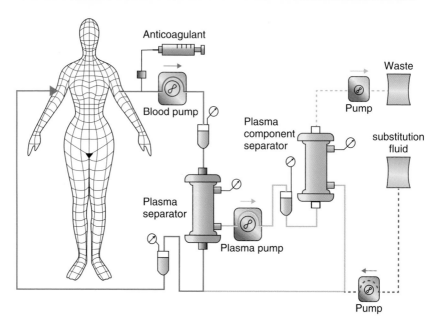

Figure 4.1 Double-filtration plasmapheresis (DFPP)

fact that it can be used in combined ABOi and HLAi transplantation, as described later.

Specific immunoabsorption is performed using the Glycorex column; this consists of a carbohydrate moiety bound to a sepharose matrix, which will absorb anti-A, anti-B, or both anti-A and anti-B isohemagglutinins [18], with a median reduction of 81% for IgG and 56% for IgM [19]. The column appears to be highly specific, with minimal effect on other proteins (including HLA antibody) and in particular coagulation factors; there is evidence that antibodies to some pneumococcal and hemophilus antigens are reduced, possibly due to a crossreactive effect, while antitetanus and antidiphtheria antibodies are unaffected [19]. Although there is significant patient variability, a reduction by approximately one or two dilutions may be achieved after each treatment. The significant difficulty with this column is the fact that it is only licensed for single use, making it a relatively expensive treatment. However, it can be incorporated into a tailored protocol, as described later.

The aim of antibody removal is to ensure that titers are sufficiently low to enable transplantation to take place without the occurrence of hyperacute rejection. Perhaps surprisingly, there is only anecdotal evidence regarding the appropriate levels immediately prior to transplantation, and indeed given the variation in reported levels from the same sample in different laboratories, it is difficult to be certain about absolute parameters. However, most centers would accept titer levels of 1 in 8 for A_1 donors and 1 in 16 for A_2. For group-B donors, some centers would accept 1 in 16, while others would require 1 in 8; at Guy's Hospital we use the latter. It should be noted that autoantibody can cause spuriously high results, and we have reported a technique to allow accurate assessment to take place despite apparently high levels of anti-A titers [20].

Recently, a new specific immunoabsorption column has appeared on the market, the Adsopak column. This contains a synthetic oligosaccharide bound to an agarose matrix, and will selectively remove anti-A or anti-B antibody. The advantage is that the column can be reused, making it relatively cost-effective. However, so far data on efficacy are limited.

Typically, two and a half to three plasma volumes are processed in one session of immunoabsorption. It should be noted that rebound of antibodies after either DFPP or immunoabsorption is common; within 12 hours, this may be due to release of tissue-bound antibody and antibody from the lymphatic and interstitial compartments, while a later rise (after 7 days) would be related to increased antibody production [15]. For these reasons, it is important to measure antibody titers on the day of transplantation, and to consider strategies for antibody suppression.

Antibody suppression
Splenectomy and rituximab
In the 1980s and 1990s, most ABOi was carried out in Japan, due to the lack of deceased donors there, and the protocols used in these cases most commonly involved splenectomy. The rationale was that removal of the spleen resulted in debulking of the B-cell population and thus reduced subsequent antibody production. The results from these series were very good when compared with compatible transplants from the same era, with graft survival rates of 84% at 1 year [21]. In theory, concomitant splenectomy carries increased risks due to the additional surgical procedure and the subsequent risk of infection from encapsulated bacteria, although in practice this does not seem to have been a major problem in Japan [22].

Splenectomy was replaced as a therapeutic strategy when Tyden, in his landmark paper [18], described four ABOi carried out using rituximab as a "chemical splenectomy." Rituximab is an anti-CD20 chimeric mouse/human antibody that results in rapid depletion of CD20-positive B cells via antibody-dependent cell-mediated cytotoxicity. B-cell counts fall effectively to zero within 2 weeks of administration, and take 12 months to recover after a single dose [23]. It should be noted that B cells in the peripheral blood account for only a small proportion of the total B-cell population, and rituximab has been shown to reduce B cells in both lymph nodes [23] and the spleen [24]. Current regimens for ABOi include a single dose of rituximab given 1 month prior to transplantation. There is no evidence that this results in any short-term reduction in antibody, and indeed one would not expect this to be the case, since long-lived plasma-cell clones would continue to produce antibody for months, or possibly years. It may be, however, that B-cell elimination has significant effects due to the actions of B-cells as antigen-presenting cells and in cytokine production [25]. The conventional dose of rituximab used is 375 mg/m², but some have experimented with lower doses with good results [26]. The Johns Hopkins group has dispensed with rituximab altogether, and recently reported outcomes in 28 patients [27]. However, they used both pre- and post-transplant plasmapheresis and intravenous immunoglobulin (IVIG), and there were five clinical and three subclinical cases of antibody-mediated rejection (AMR). Another center has achieved excellent results in a study of 37 patients, although two had AMR [28]. A recent study suggested that when compared with splenectomy, the use of rituximab resulted in lower rates of acute AMR after ABOi (although this was not statistically significant) [29]. At present, there is no convincing evidence that rituximab can be omitted routinely, although we have performed ABOi without it in selected cases, as described later.

IVIG

IVIG, which consists of pooled immunoglobulin from healthy volunteers, has formed an integral part of many ABOi regimens. The Swedish group originally described using a small dose (0.5 g/kg) on the day prior to transplantation [30], and many other centers now use this approach. The effects of IVIG are incompletely understood but may be due to a combination of an anti-idiotypic effect, downregulation of antibody production (due to an increase in circulating antibody, which is particularly important after antibody removal), interference with complement and cytokine production, and effects on the activation of T and B cells [31]. In the UK, it is expensive and difficult to source, and we have removed it from our protocol with excellent results, as described later.

Post-transplant antibody removal

Modern ABOi regimens have typically included routine post-transplant antibody removal using immunoabsorption or plasma exchange for the first week [27,30]. However, more recently the group in Freiburg developed a protocol which calls for post-transplant removal only if titers rise [32]. Thresholds for intervention were 1 in 8 in the first week and 1 in 16 in the second week, and 7 of 22 patients required post-transplant intervention.

In our own protocol at Guy's Hospital, we have abandoned routine postoperative antibody removal (after the first nine patients in the program). We intervene if there is a rise of two titer dilutions or more postoperatively, or a rise associated with biopsy-proven rejection. In 67 patients, we have only carried out "on-demand" postoperative removal on four occasions, with a good response in each case.

Accommodation

"Accommodation" has been defined as the absence of graft dysfunction in the presence of circulating antidonor antibody—clearly this could be a hemagglutinin or an HLA antibody. After ABOi, hemagglutinin titers usually remain low, but the antibody is still detectable, despite normal graft function. Given the fact that titers fall immediately post-transplantation and remain low despite—in most cases—no further treatment, it seems likely that at least part of this fall simply represents binding of antibody to the allograft with subsequent depletion of the circulating pool. Additional evidence for this comes from the fact that the majority of ABOi recipients will have positive C4d staining on biopsy, without graft dysfunction [33–35], implying that complement activation occurs as a result of antibody binding to the endothelial cell. However, it may also be the case that downregulation of antibody production occurs in the longer term, and there is additional evidence of downregulation of blood-group antigen expression on the endothelial cell surface after ABOi [36]. Although data are limited, it would seem that initial concerns that circulating antibody could lead to the development of transplant glomerulopathy and impaired graft function are not borne out [35]. In summary, accommodation does seem to occur in ABOi, but the mechanisms are poorly understood, and further research is clearly needed.

Outcomes after ABOi

As noted earlier, there are a number of different protocols currently being used in ABOi, including standard- and reduced-dose rituximab and IVIG, as well as plasmapheresis or immunoabsorption pre- and possibly postoperatively. For this reason, accurate comparisons of outcomes after ABOi are difficult. However, it is fair to say that there is good evidence that short-term outcomes are excellent, and broadly comparable with blood-group-compatible transplants. Table 4.3 shows results from all studies with

Table 4.3 Short-term outcomes of ABOi.

Author	N	Regimen	Death Censored Graft survival	Rejection
Takahashi 2006	564	Variable: included splenectomy	86% at 1 year	42% at 3 months
Tyden 2007	60	R, IA, Triple therapy	97% at mean 18 months	N/A
Ishida 2007	117	Splenectomy, DFPP, Triple therapy	94% at 1 year	15% at 6 months
Montgomery 2009	60	Variable: included post-op PE	98% at 1 year, 89% at 5 years	35%
Toki 2010	57	Variable: included splenectomy	93% at 3 years	33% AMR at 3 months
Flint 2011	37	DFPP +ivIg, pre and post-op Triple therapy	10% at 26 months	22% at 26 months
Lawrence 2011	56	R or A, DFPP, Triple therapy	98% at 1 year	18% at 1 year
Mamode 2011	54	R, DFPP or IA, Triple therapy	97% at 2 years	27% at 2 years

R = Rituximab, A = Alemtuzimab, PE = plasma exchange, IA = Immunoabsorption, Triple therapy = Tacrolimus, MMF, Prednisolone

Table 4.4 Long-term outcomes of ABOi.

Author	N	Regimen	Death Censored Graft survival	Rejection
Wilpert 2010	40	R, Ivig, Triple therapy	100 % at 39 months	28%
Tanabe 1998	67	Irradiation, splenectomy, DSG, ALG, Cya, aza, prenisolone	73% at 8 years	N/A
Takahashi 2006	564	Variable, including splenectomy	74% at 5 years and 53% at 10 years	
Ishida 2007	117	Splenectomy, DFPP, Tri[le therapy	90% at 5 years	N/A

DSG= deoxyspergualin, ALG= anti-lymphocyte globulin, Cya= cyclosporine, aza=azathioprine

over 30 patients reporting outcomes over the last 10 years [22,27,28,37–40], and includes our own data [41]. What is clear from these data is that outcomes after ABOi in the short term are excellent, although they mostly come from small, single-center studies. Longer-term studies are less common (see Table 4.4) but also show excellent outcomes [5,42]. These include a large series from Japan [21].

A key question is whether all patients undergoing ABOi are likely to have the same outcomes or whether baseline hemagglutinnin titers will affect success rates. In our own experience, we have never failed to reduce titers adequately, despite baseline titers of 1 in 1024 in some cases, and indeed some centers in Japan do not have an upper limit of baseline titer in consideration for transplantation. There are however some caveats: we have had to carry out repeated attempts (on separate occasions) in a single patient, which is costly and psychologically difficult for both recipient and donor. Furthermore, when repeated sessions of antibody removal are performed, the patient will become physically exhausted and edematous, even when immunoabsorption rather than plasmapheresis is used. There is conflicting evidence regarding the likelihood of poorer outcomes with higher baseline titers; some have suggested that outcome does depend on baseline titer [43], while others have found no association [37,44]. Our approach has been to avoid attempting ABOi in patients with titers above 1 in 1024; for those with titers of 1 in 512 or 1 in 1024, we may suggest one or two runs in the UK paired scheme prior to ABOi, depending on patient preference. All other patients are offered ABOi, but can opt for one or more runs in the paired scheme first if they wish.

Pediatric ABOi
Very few ABOi transplants have been performed in children. This is partly due to concerns about the stronger immune response in the young, and partly to the prioritization of children in many deceased-donor allocation

Table 4.5 Reported outcomes after pediatric blood-group-incompatible transplantation.

Author and year	No.	Therapy	Outcomes	Rejection	Follow-up (months)
Ohta 2000	10	Splenectomy, ALG, Pex	100% GS	6 patients (1 hyperacute)	65 (Median)
Shishido 2001	16	Splenectomy ALG, cyclophosphamide, Pex/IA	1 year GS 87%, 5 year GS	1 hyperacute	63 (Mean)
Genberg 2008/2010	9	Rituximab, IA	100% GS	Nil	> 12
Mamode 2012	5	Rituximab, IA/DFPP	100% GS	1 (non-compliance)	29 (Mean)

schemes, meaning that waiting times are usually short. Countries with little or no deceased donation, such as Japan, have had the most active pediatric ABOi programs [45–47], although these groups have used aggressive immunosuppressive regimens, including splenectomy and antilymphocyte globulin. Tyden's group in Sweden has performed eight cases, with 100% graft survival and no rejection [48,49], and in the UK we have carried out five cases (two in Newcastle, three at Guy's/Great Ormond Street Hospitals) [50], again with excellent results. The largest study to date—from Japan—reports the outcomes in 111 children undergoing ABOi, mostly using splenectomy [51]. Graft survival was 96% at 1 year and 86% at 5 years, and interestingly these outcomes were superior to those after ABOi in adults. There was no post-transplant lymphoproliferative disorder (PTLD). These studies are summarized in Table 4.5.

It is clear from these early data that high rates of rejection or poor graft survival have not been evident in pediatric ABOi. However, experience is currently limited to a low number of small, single-center studies, and clearly we require more substantial data before it is possible to determine how pediatric ABOi compares with blood-group-compatible living-donor or indeed deceased-donor transplantation.

A protocol for ABOi

We describe here the approach to ABOi at Guy's Hospital; as stated earlier, there are many variations, and ours may not be the most appropriate. Our philosophy has been based on tailoring therapy according to baseline titers, so that we are able to minimize perioperative immunosuppression and avoid complications. Additionally, we have opted to use immunoabsorption for antibody removal (with Glycorex or TheraSorb columns) unless baseline titers are low, in which case we use DFPP. The aim of this approach is to minimize problems arising from coagulopathy and hypoalbuminemia arising from repeated sessions of DFPP.

A summary of our approach is shown in Figure 4.2. Essentially, for patients with the lowest baseline titers (<1 in 8), we avoid any additional treatment; patients are given the same regimen as a standard living-donor

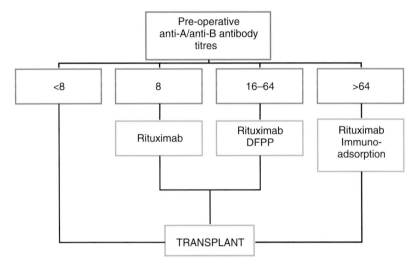

Figure 4.2 Guy's Hospital algorithm for ABOi

transplant. At levels of 1 in 8, we simply use a preoperative dose of rituximab, but no antibody removal. For titers between 1 in 16 and 1 in 64 (inclusive), we use rituximab and preoperative DFPP only. For titers above 1 in 64, we use rituximab and preoperative immunoabsorption with Glycorex or TheraSorb columns. We abandoned routine postoperative antibody removal and preoperative IVIG after the first nine patients. All patients are given basiliximab induction, tacrolimus (initial levels of 10–12 ng/ml), mycophenylate mofetil 2 g/day (commenced 1 week preoperatively), and prednisolone (with a steroid wean at 6 months if there is no rejection). So far, 80 patients have been transplanted; we recently reported results from the first 54, with a 2-year graft-survival rate of 97%, compared with 99% for a control group of 139 compatible patients transplanted during the same period (p = 0.750). T-cell-mediated rejection rates were similar in both groups (27 versus 18%), while AMR rates were 8% in ABOi and 3% in controls, although this was not significantly different [41].

In summary, tailoring the protocol according to baseline titers can produce excellent results and avoid overimmunosuppression and excess costs.

Alternatives to ABOi

For those presenting with a blood-group-incompatible donor, assuming there are no available compatible living donors, there are essentially three alternatives: remain on the deceased-donor list, enter a paired-exchange or pooled scheme, or undergo ABOi. Our approach has been to always consider a blood-group-compatible transplant if possible, despite the excellent results from ABOi. However, if there are no compatible donors, we prefer ABOi over listing for deceased donation, unless baseline hemagglutinin titers are over 1 in 1024. All patients are offered the option of entering the paired scheme, but again, for those with high titers this is the preferred option.

Table 4.6 Number of transplants against numbers of registered recipients in the UK paired-exchange scheme according to original donor and recipient blood groups.

Donor blood group	Recipient blood group			
	O	A	B	AB
O	15/114	21/42	6/22	0/1
	(13%)	(50%)	(27%)	(0%)
A	23/152	12/54	11/33	0/3
	(15%)	(22%)	(33%)	(0%)
B	6/47	10/28	0/18	1/3
	(13%)	(36%)	(0%)	(33%)
AB	0/7	0/4	0/6	0/1
	(0%)	(0%)	(0%)	(0%)

courtesy R Johnson NHSBT, private correspondence 2011.

Increasingly, data are becoming available regarding the likelihood of successful matching in the paired scheme. The frequency of blood groups shown in Table 4.1 clearly indicates that the most common blood-group incompatibility is A into O. In this pairing, the recipient would need to be matched with a group-O donor, but more importantly their own donor would be seeking a group-A recipient. Clearly, an O-into-A pairing would only be entered into the paired scheme due to HLA incompatibility, and these antibodies could then preclude transplantation from the new A donor; in 2011 in the UK, 73% of 163 potential recipients registered for paired exchange had a calculated reaction frequency of 85% or higher, meaning that that they would have had a positive crossmatch against 85% or more of the last 10 000 deceased donors. Table 4.6 shows transplants performed through the UK paired-exchange scheme according to the blood groups of the original pair. Thus, for the most common incompatibility, A into O, only 15% have obtained a transplant, with a similar figure for B into O. A-into-B or B-into-A pairings are more successful, with around a third receiving a transplant, but for AB donors the situation is dismal, with no successful transplants recorded. Similar findings have been reported by the Johns Hopkins group from North American paired-exchange schemes [7].

For A- or B-into-O pairings, our advice to patients is that the chance of success in the paired scheme is a little more than 1 in 10. Certainly if such a pairing has not achieved a successful match after several runs, the probability of a subsequent match dramatically decreases, since only a small number of new pairs enter the scheme each year. For such incompatible pairs, antibody removal should be considered.

Variations on paired-exchange schemes may help such pairs; voluntary entry of antibody-compatible pairs into a paired scheme has been explored in the USA [7] and is due to be introduced in the UK in 2012. Currently it remains to be seen whether this will make a significant impact on matching for blood-group-incompatible pairs.

Finally, a new approach to blood-group-incompatible deceased-donor transplantation has been proposed. We have shown that 45% of children on the UK waiting list could accept a blood-group-incompatible transplant, since their hemagglutinin titers are 1 in 16 or less, meaning that a single preoperative session of antibody removal, or none at all, would allow ABOi to proceed [52]. Modeling of the effect of introducing a policy of listing these children for deceased-donor ABOi suggests that mean waiting times would be reduced and there would be a 2% increase in pediatric transplants.

HLA-incompatible transplantation

Donor-specific HLA antibodies (DSAs) are not normally present, but typically are thought to arise from three sources: previous transplantation, pregnancy, or blood transfusion. They may lead to a positive flow or complement-dependent cytotoxicity (CDC) crossmatch—where transplantation is usually impossible without antibody removal—or they may cause early aggressive humoral rejection, even after removal. This typically occurs around 2 weeks after transplantation, and is thought to be due to immune memory, with activation of B- and T-cell clones. In contrast to ABOi, outcomes are significantly poorer than compatible transplants, and complication rates are high [53]. Inferior graft survival reflects both aggressive acute rejection and an increased incidence of chronic AMR, which is now thought to be the major cause of graft loss [54]. This section considers approaches to antibody measurement and removal, perioperative issues, outcomes from HLAi, and recent developments.

Measurement of donor-specific HLA antibody

Recent technological advances have meant that it is now relatively easy to measure DSAs, using so-called solid-phase techniques, where soluble or recombinant HLA molecules are combined with a solid matrix then tested against serum. These include the enzyme-linked immunosorbent assay (ELISA) technique, flow-cytometric analysis (both of which are semi-quantitative), and the Luminex system (which provides a quantitative read-out for individual HLA antibodies). In the Luminex system, microparticles are coated with specific HLAs so that HLA antibody within the serum will bind and can be detected by the addition of antihuman IgG, which causes fluorescence. This results in a read-out that gives a mean fluorescence index (MFI) for each DSA, as shown in Figure 4.3. Thresholds for denoting DSAs as "positive" are arbitrary, vary between different centers, and are not evidence-based. Typically, individual DSAs are combined to give a total MFI value, although this presupposes equivalent affinity for each antibody, which may not be the case. There are two important concepts to consider when assessing antibody levels: first, binding is dependent on the antigenic moiety that the antibody "sees." This antigenic "epitope" is formed from the three-dimensional configuration of the HLA protein on the endothelial

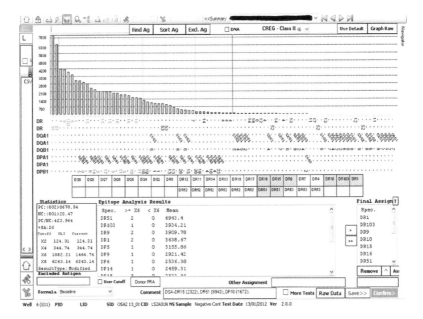

Figure 4.3 HLA-antibody profile derived from Luminex

cell surface. This structure may be bound by more than one antibody, and antibody binding may vary between epitopes or even with different antibodies for the same epitope. The importance of these facts is that the presence of a DSA in itself is not the only important issue—it is the combination of both the amount of antibody and the avidity for the antigen which will determine the significance.

The second issue is that antibody is not an infallible read-out for immune memory. Thus there may be memory B cells against a particular HLA antigen despite relatively low circulating antibody; exposure to the antigen may then generate a response with production of vast quantities of antibody and graft destruction. A similar concept may apply to the relationship between memory T cells and antibody levels, although this has not yet been comprehensively demonstrated. The implication of this concept is that reexposure to HLA antigen is important, even when circulating antibody levels are low: this is termed a repeat mismatch, and outcomes relative to this are discussed later. Clearly, it is usually possible to predict repeat mismatches where previous exposure has arisen from a transplant, or even from pregnancy, assuming histocompatibility typing is available for the father, but this is not possible where sensitization occurs as a result of blood transfusion.

The second method of assessment in HLAi is the crossmatch. Previously, the CDC crossmatch—based on the ability of antibodies in recipient sera to induce cell lysis in donor lymphoytes in the presence of (rabbit) complement—was used routinely, but this has been superseded by the flow-cytometric crossmatch in many centers. The CDC crossmatch is relatively crude, does not account for non-complement-fixing antibodies, and can be misinterpreted when IgM autoreactive antibodies, which may result in a "false-positive" crossmatch, are present. The flow crossmatch is more sensitive than a CDC crossmatch, although individual centers may consider transplanting across a weakly positive flow crossmatch in selected cases. The flow crossmatch may be performed as a titer crossmatch for T and B cells separately, so that a result is expressed as an antibody dilution, as with hemagglutinin titers (e.g. T-cell crossmatch positive at 1 in 4); alternatively, relative mean immunofluorescence (RMF) may be used (in our laboratory an RMF of 2.35 is considered indicative of a positive crossmatch). In some centers, this is expressed as mean channel shift, with a cut-off of 150–300 being considered positive.

Recently, the virtual crossmatch has become widely used [10,55]. This involves predicting a negative crossmatch from the donor antigen and recipient antibody profiles, without the need to actually perform a crossmatch. This may be effectively put in place through an organ-allocation scheme or may be used by individual centers to decrease cold-ischemic time.

Non-HLA antibodies

In addition to class I and II HLA antibodies, it has become increasingly apparent in recent years that other antibodies may lead to acute AMR. These are often termed "anti-endothelial-cell antibodies," as the antigens may not appear on peripheral blood lymphocytes, and include anti-MICA (major histocompatibility complex class I-related A) [56] and GSTT1 antibodies, but currently evidence regarding the importance of these is limited, and hampered by the lack of standardized assays [57].

HLA-antibody removal

The options for antibody removal are similar to those described for ABOi. Splenectomy was previously performed routinely before transplantation by some groups, but has now fallen out of favor, with its main role today being that of rescue therapy postoperatively in severe AMR [58]. Thus the main options are immunoabsorption, using nonspecific columns such as TheraSorb, and plasmapheresis, with the aim of achieving a negative crossmatch prior to surgery. Both methods have already been described in detail. Currently, no HLA-specific immunoabsorption columns are available, although these are expected on the market soon.

HLA-antibody suppression

The main pharmacological interventions used for highly sensitized transplant recipients are anti-CD20 antibody (rituximab) and IVIG. Both have already been described in detail but there are some issues specific to HLAi. Administration of rituximab will lead to subsequent difficulties with a B-cell crossmatch, as the antibody will bind to donor B cells. Clearly, in HLAi, close monitoring of the crossmatch immediately prior to transplantation is important in order to avoid accelerated acute rejection. Rituximab can be cleaved using pronase, but this is a time-consuming process. In our own laboratory, if rituximab is used before transplantation we perform a final B-cell crossmatch immediately prior to administration, and subsequently use Luminex beads to monitor HLA antibody, using MFI levels to determine whether it is safe to proceed to transplantation.

Several centers have reported outcomes after the use of rituximab in HLAi [59], but some do not routinely use it, including our own. Currently there are no randomized trials of the use of anti-CD20 antibody before HLAi transplantation. However, it has been used in conjunction with high-dose IVIG (2 g/kg) to reduce HLA antibody in highly sensitized patients and allow successful deceased-donor transplantation [60].

IVIG is also used as part of an induction protocol in HLAi. In this situation, 0.5 g/kg is typically given, either as a single dose prior to surgery or in repeated doses after each plasmapheresis. The rationale for the latter is that restoration of circulating-antibody levels prevents the rebound production of antibody after removal.

Perioperative issues in HLAi
Even when antibody is removed in order to achieve a negative crossmatch at the time of transplantation, HLAi remains an immunologically high-risk procedure. This risk is increased when there is a repeat mismatch. For this reason, the use of more potent induction agents has been advocated. Although there are no randomized trials in highly sensitized patients, the use of ATG and alemtuzumab has been shown to be beneficial in those at higher immunological risk; in our own practice, we use the latter.

The risk of bleeding is increased in those undergoing antibody removal, although it is lessened with the use of immunoabsorption columns. Relaparotomy for bleeding is not uncommon, and close monitoring of clotting factors in the perioperative period is vital. As noted earlier, we administer fibrinogen preoperatively if the level is less than 1 g/l on the day of surgery.

It is clear from our experience that many patients undergoing HLAi have increased comorbidities, which may be related to longstanding renal failure (they may have a previous transplant) or a long wait on the deceased-donor list. The addition of antibody-removal therapy (which may induce hypoproteinemia and can leave patients physically exhausted), the use of stronger induction therapies, and the risk of perioperative bleeding combine to dramatically increase the risk of complications after transplantation. For this reason, our approach is to carefully select patients for HLAi, with thorough investigation including a cardiac stress test, and avoid transplantation in those whose physical condition is not robust.

Guy's hospital protocol for HLAi
Our current protocol is as follows: a test DFPP is performed to determine whether antibody removal is feasible and to predict the number of sessions required to achieve a negative flow-cytometric crossmatch. Tacrolimus and mycophenylate mofetil are commenced 1 week prior to transplantation, and daily DFPP is undertaken as required. A single dose of 0.5 g/kg IVIG is given the evening before transplantation, and a final assessment of DSA is performed on the day of surgery, using the Luminex system. Alemtuzumab

is given for induction, and tacrolimus, mycophenylate, and prednisolone are continued postoperatively. DSA levels are monitored postoperatively, but antibody removal is not performed unless levels rise or there is associated acute AMR.

Outcomes after HLAi

It is widely accepted that outcomes after HLAi are inferior to those in conventional living donation. However, an important recent publication [61], which analyzed US registry data, has clearly shown that patient survival is superior in those undergoing HLAi when compared with those who remain on the deceased-donor list in the hope of receiving a compatible deceased-donor organ (81 versus 66% patient survival at 5 years, $p < 0.001$).

Outcome data from other studies are limited; these are largely single-center, low-volume studies from centers with expertise in HLAi, and often the definition of HLAi varies. However, if we consider recent studies of patients with a positive flow or CDC crossmatch, 1-year graft-survival rates range from 82 to 96% [60,62–65]. Long-term survival data are even more limited, although one study of 41 patients showed a 69% 5-year survival [53]. It is difficult to extrapolate these results more widely, but in addition to these data, analysis of the UK registry (which has a mandatory requirement for all transplants to be registered) shows graft-survival rates in 109 HLAi to be 87% at 3 years, although 22% of these had a negative crossmatch but positive DSA [66]. In summary, graft survival after HLAi is probably inferior to that from compatible living-donor transplantation, but it would seem reasonable to expect an overall 1-year graft survival rate of around 85%.

A key concern is that late graft loss will be increased due to chronic AMR in the context of persistent donor-specific antibody. The incidence of transplant glomerulopathy and interstitial fibrosis and tubular atrophy (IFTA) is increased after HLAi [67], and long-term graft survival is inferior to that with antibody-compatible transplants, but as noted earlier, outcomes are better than remaining on the deceased-donor list [61].

Alternatives to HLAi

As with ABOi, alternatives include remaining on the deceased-donor list or entering an exchange scheme. Transplantation via the exchange scheme offers the possibility of an antibody-compatible transplant, which would have lower risks and better long-term graft survival. The earlier comments regarding blood-group incompatibility and the chance of success after repeated runs in a paired scheme apply equally to HLA incompatibility, but if there is blood-group compatibility or a group-O donor it is certainly true that two or three runs in the paired-exchange scheme would be preferable to HLAi unless the crossmatch is only a borderline positive with no repeat mismatches. Our own policy is to offer patients the paired scheme first and proceed to HLAi if they are unsuccessful after two or more runs.

The recent data from the USA have shown clearly that HLAi is preferable to remaining on the deceased-donor waiting list in that country [61], and while this may not be universally applicable (for example, where deceased-donor rates are higher, such as in Spain), with careful selection of patients HLAi should be considered appropriate when an exchange scheme has failed to secure a transplant.

New developments in antibody-incompatible transplantation

The excellent results reported after ABOi might suggest that there is little room for improvement. However, it remains difficult to transplant patients with high baseline hemagglutinin titers. An interesting approach which might help involves using a recombinant endogalactosidase to effectively deplete A or B antigen on baboon kidney and liver cells, using an in vivo infusion [68]. Furthermore, the ability to reproduce the effect using ex vivo perfusion and cold storage in the same experiment offers exciting potential for deceased-donor ABOi transplantation.

In HLAi, a major problem is the high rate of rejection, and in particular AMR. Recently the Mayo Clinic group has used a new monoclonal antibody, eculizumab, to prevent this [69]. Eculizumab inhibits the formation of the C5a-9 membrane attack complex, which is one of the final mechanisms by which antibody provokes disruption of the endothelial cell. Eculizumab was used as part of a protocol for HLAi, in which it was given for several weeks after transplantation in an attempt to prevent AMR. Of 26 patients, two sustained AMR (7%), which is much lower than the expected rate of around 40%. Currently a multicenter phase II trial is underway to test the concept.

Another potentially useful new agent is bortezomib, a proteasome inhibitor which depletes plasma cells. This drug has been used both prior to transplantation, in an attempt to reduce antibody, and after transplantation, to treat AMR. Currently the evidence for efficacy in either setting is limited [70–72], which may be due to the fact that complete depletion of plasma cells does not occur and indeed is undesirable. Nevertheless, bortezomib may find a niche within the HLAi as more data become available.

Finally, human studies of new B-cell-depleting agents are waited with interest.

Conclusion: what should we do with an antibody-incompatible recipient?

AIT is a rapidly developing field and involves an increasingly large proportion of the transplant population. Good evidence for specific therapeutic options is limited. However, the following is based on a combination of existing evidence and experience, and represents one (but not necessarily a definitive) approach.

For ABOi, if baseline titers are extremely high (>1 in 1024), deceased donation and/or the paired scheme is appropriate. For those with lower titers, consideration can be given to antibody removal and direct incompatible transplantation. If patient or clinician preference is to exhaust all options first, it would be reasonable to enter a paired-exchange scheme, bearing in mind the likely chance of a match. After two or three runs in a scheme, further runs are unlikely to have a positive result. For those with low baseline hemaglutinnins (1 in 32 or less), direct ABOi is the preferred option. Pediatric patients can also undergo successful ABOi.

For HLAi, attempts should be made to risk-stratify patients, based on baseline DSA levels and crossmatch titers, the presence of repeat mismatches, and the degree of antibody reduction after test removal. Immunological risk should be balanced against the increased perioperative risks, and HLAi in frail patients at high risk of rejection should be avoided. Again, a paired-exchange scheme and waiting for a deceased donor remain options, but they should not be pursued indefinitely in those who are able to undergo more aggressive treatments.

References

1 Hume DM, Merrill JP, Miller BF, Thorn GW. Experiences with renal homotransplantation in the human: report of nine cases. *The Journal of Clinical Investigation* 1955;34(2):327–382.

2 Terasaki PI, Mickey MR, Singal DP, Mittal KK, Patel R. Serotyping for homotransplantation. *XX. Selection of recipients for cadaver donor transplants. The New England Journal of Medicine* 1968;279(20):1101–1103.

3 Alexandre GP, Squifflet JP, De Bruyere M, Latinne D, Reding R, Gianello P, et al. Present experiences in a series of 26 ABO-incompatible living donor renal allografts. *Transplantation Proceedings* 1987;19(6):4538–4542.

4 Palmer A, Taube D, Welsh K, Bewick M, Gjorstrup P, Thick M. Removal of anti-HLA antibodies by extracorporeal immunoadsorption to enable renal transplantation. *Lancet* 1989;1(8628):10–12.

5 Tanabe K, Takahashi K, Sonda K, Tokumoto T, Ishikawa N, Kawai T, et al. Long-term results of ABO-incompatible living kidney transplantation: a single-center experience. *Transplantation* 1998;65(2):224–228.

6 Reisaeter AV, Leivestad T, Albrechtsen D, Holdaas H, Hartmann A, Sodal G, et al. Pretransplant plasma exchange or immunoadsorption facilitates renal transplantation in immunized patients. *Transplantation* 1995;60(3):242–248.

7 Montgomery RA. Renal transplantation across HLA and ABO antibody barriers: integrating paired donation into desensitization protocols. *American journal of transplantation: official journal of the American Society of Transplantation and the American Society of Transplant Surgeons* 2010;10(3):449–457.

8 Segev DL, Gentry SE, Warren DS, Reeb B, Montgomery RA. Kidney paired donation and optimizing the use of live donor organs. *JAMA* 2005;293(15): 1883–1890.

9 Roodnat JI, Kal-van Gestel JA, Zuidema W, van Noord MA, van de Wetering J, JN IJ, et al. Successful expansion of the living donor pool by alternative living donation programs. *American Journal of Transplantation* 2009;9(9): 2150–2156.

10 Fuggle SV, Martin S. Tools for human leukocyte antigen antibody detection and their application to transplanting sensitized patients. *Transplantation* 2008; 86(3):384–390.

11 Rydberg L. ABO-incompatibility in solid organ transplantation. *Transfus Med* 2001;11(4):325–342.

12 Nelson PW, Landreneau MD, Luger AM, Pierce GE, Ross G, Shield CF, 3rd,, *et al.* Ten-year experience in transplantation of A2 kidneys into B and O recipients. *Transplantation* 1998;65(2):256–260.

13 Kumlien G, Wilpert J, Safwenberg J, Tyden G. Comparing the tube and gel techniques for ABO antibody titration, as performed in three European centers. *Transplantation* 2007;84(12 Suppl):S17–S19.

14 Krishnan NS, Fleetwood P, Higgins RM, Hathaway M, Zehnder D, Mitchell D, *et al.* Application of flow cytometry to monitor antibody levels in ABO incompatible kidney transplantation. *Transplantation* 2008;86(3):474–477.

15 Schwenger V, Morath C. Immunoadsorption in nephrology and kidney transplantation. *Nephrology, Dialysis, Transplantation* 2010;25(8):2407–2413.

16 Matic G, Hofmann D, Winkler R, Tiess M, Michelsen A, Schneidewind JM, *et al.* Removal of immunoglobulins by a protein A versus an antihuman immunoglobulin G-based system: evaluation of 602 sessions of extracorporeal immunoadsorption. *Artificial Organs* 2000;24(2):103–107.

17 Staudt A, Bohm M, Knebel F, Grosse Y, Bischoff C, Hummel A, *et al.* Potential role of autoantibodies belonging to the immunoglobulin G-3 subclass in cardiac dysfunction among patients with dilated cardiomyopathy. *Circulation* 2002;106(19):2448–2453.

18 Tyden G, Kumlien G, Fehrman I. Successful ABO-incompatible kidney trans-plantations without splenectomy using antigen-specific immunoadsorption and rituximab. *Transplantation* 2003;76(4):730–731.

19 Valli PV, Puga Yung G, Fehr T, Schulz-Huotari C, Kaup N, Gungor T, *et al. Changes of circulating antibody levels induced by ABO antibody adsorption for ABO-incompatible kidney transplantation. American Journal of Transplantation* 2009;9(5):1072–1080.

20 Barnett N, Nightingale A, Maggs T, Needs M, Williams E, Curran D, *et al.* High anti-A titres may not preclude ABO-incompatible renal transplantation: an autoantibody could be the culprit. *Nephrology, Dialysis, Transplantation* 2010;25(11):3794–3796.

21 Takahashi K, Saito K, Takahara S, Okuyama A, Tanabe K, Toma H, *et al.* Excel-lent long-term outcome of ABO-incompatible living donor kidney transplan-tation in Japan. *American Journal of Transplantation* 2004;4(7):1089–1096.

22 Takahashi K, Saito K. Present status of ABO-incompatible kidney transplan-tation in Japan. *Xenotransplantation* 2006;13(2):118–122.

23 Genberg H, Hansson A, Wernerson A, Wennberg L, Tyden G. Pharmaco-dynamics of rituximab in kidney allotransplantation. *American Journal of Transplantation* 2006;6(10):2418–2428.

24 Toki D, Ishida H, Horita S, Setoguchi K, Yamaguchi Y, Tanabe K. Impact of low-dose rituximab on splenic B cells in ABO-incompatible renal transplant recipients. *Transplant International* 2009;22(4):447–454.

25 Barnett N, Dorling A, Mamode N. B cells in renal transplantation: pathological aspects and therapeutic interventions. *Nephrology, Dialysis, Transplantation* 2011;26(3):767–774.

26 Shirakawa H, Ishida H, Shimizu T, Omoto K, Iida S, Toki D, *et al.* The low dose of rituximab in ABO-incompatible kidney transplantation without a splenectomy: a single-center experience. *Clinical Transplantation* 2011;25(6): 878–884.

27 Montgomery RA, Locke JE, King KE, Segev DL, Warren DS, Kraus ES, *et al.* ABO incompatible renal transplantation: a paradigm ready for broad implementation. *Transplantation* 2009;87(8):1246–1255.

28 Flint SM, Walker RG, Hogan C, Haeusler MN, Robertson A, Francis DM, *et al.* Successful ABO-incompatible kidney transplantation with antibody removal and standard immunosuppression. *American Journal of Transplantation* 2011;11(5):1016–1024.

29 Fuchinoue S, Ishii Y, Sawada T, Murakami T, Iwadoh K, Sannomiya A, *et al.* The 5-year outcome of ABO-incompatible kidney transplantation with rituximab induction. *Transplantation* 2011;91(8):853–857.

30 Tyden G, Kumlien G, Genberg H, Sandberg J, Lundgren T, Fehrman I. ABO incompatible kidney transplantations without splenectomy, using antigen-specific immunoadsorption and rituximab. *American Journal of Transplantation* 2005;5(1):145–148.

31 Negi VS, Elluru S, Siberil S, Graff-Dubois S, Mouthon L, Kazatchkine MD, *et al.* Intravenous immunoglobulin: an update on the clinical use and mechanisms of action. *Journal of Clinical Immunology* 2007;27(3):233–245.

32 Wilpert J, Geyer M, Pisarski P, Drognitz O, Schulz-Huotari C, Gropp A, *et al.* On-demand strategy as an alternative to conventionally scheduled post-transplant immunoadsorptions after ABO-incompatible kidney transplantation. *Nephrology, Dialysis, Transplantation* 2007;22(10):3048–3051.

33 Haas M, Rahman MH, Racusen LC, Kraus ES, Bagnasco SM, Segev DL, *et al.* C4d and C3d staining in biopsies of ABO- and HLA-incompatible renal allografts: correlation with histologic findings. *American Journal of Transplantation* 2006;6(8):1829–1840.

34 Gloor JM, Cosio FG, Rea DJ, Wadei HM, Winters JL, Moore SB, *et al.* Histologic findings one year after positive crossmatch or ABO blood group incompatible living donor kidney transplantation. *American Journal of Transplantation* 2006;6(8):1841–1847.

35 Setoguchi K, Ishida H, Shimmura H, Shimizu T, Shirakawa H, Omoto K, *et al.* Analysis of renal transplant protocol biopsies in ABO-incompatible kidney transplantation. *American Journal of Transplantation* 2008;8(1):86–94.

36 Tanabe T, Ishida H, Horita S, Yamaguchi Y, Toma H, Tanabe K. Decrease of blood type antigenicity over the long-term after ABO-incompatible kidney transplantation. *Transplant Immunology* 2011;25(1):1–6.

37 Toki D, Ishida H, Setoguchi K, Shimizu T, Omoto K, Shirakawa H, *et al.* Acute antibody-mediated rejection in living ABO-incompatible kidney transplantation: long-term impact and risk factors. *American Journal of Transplantation* 2009;9(3):567–577.

38 Lawrence C, Galliford JW, Willicombe MK, McLean AG, Lesabe M, Rowan F, *et al.* Antibody removal before ABO-incompatible renal transplantation: how much plasma exchange is therapeutic? *Transplantation* 2011;92(10):1129–1133.

39 Tyden G, Donauer J, Wadstrom J, Kumlien G, Wilpert J, Nilsson T, *et al.* Implementation of a protocol for ABO-incompatible kidney transplantation—a three-center experience with 60 consecutive transplantations. *Transplantation* 2007;83(9):1153–1155.

40 Ishida H, Miyamoto N, Shirakawa H, Shimizu T, Tokumoto T, Ishikawa N, *et al.* Evaluation of immunosuppressive regimens in ABO-incompatible living kidney transplantation—single center analysis. *American Journal of Transplantation* 2007;7(4):825–831.

41 Mamode N, Hadjianastassiou V, Dorling A, Kenchayikoppad S, Barnett N. Successful Outcomes after Minimising Antibody Modulation in Blood

Group Incompatible Transplantation. 2011; *Glasgow*, UK: European Society of Transplantation.

42 Wilpert J, Fischer KG, Pisarski P, Wiech T, Daskalakis M, Ziegler A, *et al.* Long-term outcome of ABO-incompatible living donor kidney transplantation based on antigen-specific desensitization. An observational comparative analysis. Nephrology, Dialysis, *Transplantation* 2010;25(11):3778–3786.

43 Shimmura H, Tanabe K, Ishikawa N, Tokumoto T, Takahashi K, Toma H. Role of anti-A/B antibody titers in results of ABO-incompatible kidney transplantation. *Transplantation* 2000;70(9):1331–1335.

44 Tobian AA, Shirey RS, Montgomery RA, Cai W, Haas M, Ness PM, *et al.* ABO antibody titer and risk of antibody-mediated rejection in ABO-incompatible renal transplantation. *American Journal of Transplantation* 2010;10(5):1247–1253.

45 Shishido S, Asanuma H, Tajima E, Hoshinaga K, Ogawa O, Hasegawa A, *et al.* ABO-incompatible living-donor kidney transplantation in children. *Transplantation* 2001;72(6):1037–1042.

46 Shishido S, Hasegawa A. Current status of ABO-incompatible kidney transplantation in children. *Pediatric Transplantation* 2005;9(2):148–1254.

47 Ohta T, Kawaguchi H, Hattori M, Takahashi K, Nagafuchi H, Akioka Y, *et al.* ABO-incompatible pediatric kidney transplantation in a single-center trial. *Pediatr Nephrol* 2000;14(1):1–5.

48 Genberg H, Kumlien G, Wennberg L, Berg U, Tyden G. ABO-incompatible kidney transplantation using antigen-specific immunoadsorption and rituximab: a 3-year follow-up. *Transplantation* 2008;85(12):1745–1754.

49 Genberg H, Kumlien G, Wennberg L, Tyden G. The efficacy of antigen-specific immunoadsorption and rebound of anti-A/B antibodies in ABO-incompatible kidney transplantation. *Nephrology, Dialysis, Transplantation* 2011;26(7):2394–2400.

50 Mamode N, Taylor J, Yse T, Marks SD. Paediatric Blood Group Incompatible Transplantation: The Initial UK Experience. 2012; *Glasgow*, UK: British Transplant Society Annual Congress.

51 Aikawa A, Takahashi K, Sato K. ABO Incompatible Pediatric Kidney Transplantation in Japan. 2011; *Montreal*, Canada: IPTA.

52 Barnett N MS, Reid C, Maggs T, Hadjianastassiou VG, Jennings C, Scanes M, Vaughan R, Mamode N. Low Titre ABO-incompatible Deceased Donor Renal Transplantation in Paediatric Patients: A New Approach to Long Waiting Lists. 2011; *Glasgow*, UK: European Society for Organ Transplantation.

53 Haririan A, Nogueira J, Kukuruga D, Schweitzer E, Hess J, Gurk-Turner C, *et al.* Positive cross-match living donor kidney transplantation: longer-term outcomes. *American Journal of Transplantation* 2009;9(3):536–542.

54 Einecke G, Sis B, Reeve J, Mengel M, Campbell PM, Hidalgo LG, *et al.* Antibody-mediated microcirculation injury is the major cause of late kidney transplant failure. *American Journal of Transplantation* 2009;9(11):2520–2531.

55 Taylor CJ, Kosmoliaptsis V, Sharples LD, Prezzi D, Morgan CH, Key T, *et al.* Ten-year experience of selective omission of the pretransplant crossmatch test in deceased donor kidney transplantation. *Transplantation* 2010;89(2):185–193.

56 Zou Y, Stastny P, Susal C, Dohler B, Opelz G. Antibodies against MICA antigens and kidney-transplant rejection. *The New England Journal of Medicine* 2007;357(13):1293–1300.

57 Regele H. Non-HLA antibodies in kidney allograft rejection: convincing concept in need of further evidence. *Kidney International* 2011;79(6):583–586.

58 Locke JE, Zachary AA, Haas M, Melancon JK, Warren DS, Simpkins CE, *et al.* The utility of splenectomy as rescue treatment for severe acute antibody mediated rejection. *American Journal of Transplantation* 2007;7(4): 842–846.

59 Becker YT, Samaniego-Picota M, Sollinger HW. The emerging role of rituximab in organ transplantation. *Transplant International* 2006;19(8): 621–628.

60 Vo AA, Lukovsky M, Toyoda M, Wang J, Reinsmoen NL, Lai CH, *et al.* Rituximab and intravenous immune globulin for desensitization during renal transplantation. *The New England Journal of Medicine* 2008;359(3):242–251.

61 Montgomery RA, Lonze BE, King KE, Kraus ES, Kucirka LM, Locke JE, *et al.* Desensitization in HLA-incompatible kidney recipients and survival. *The New England Journal of Medicine* 2011;365(4):318–326.

62 Stegall MD, Gloor J, Winters JL, Moore SB, Degoey S. A comparison of plasmapheresis versus high-dose IVIG desensitization in renal allograft recipients with high levels of donor specific alloantibody. *American Journal of Transplantation* 2006;6(2):346–351.

63 Vo AA, Wechsler EA, Wang J, Peng A, Toyoda M, Lukovsky M, *et al.* Analysis of subcutaneous (SQ) alemtuzumab induction therapy in highly sensitized patients desensitized with IVIG and rituximab. *American Journal of Transplantation* 2008;8(1):144–149.

64 Vo AA, Toyoda M, Peng A, Bunnapradist S, Lukovsky M, Jordan SC. Effect of induction therapy protocols on transplant outcomes in crossmatch positive renal allograft recipients desensitized with IVIG. *American Journal of Transplantation* 2006;6(10):2384–2390.

65 Jordan SC, Vo A, Bunnapradist S, Toyoda M, Peng A, Puliyanda D, *et al.* Intravenous immune globulin treatment inhibits crossmatch positivity and allows for successful transplantation of incompatible organs in living-donor and cadaver recipients. *Transplantation* 2003;76(4):631–636.

66 Higgins RM JR, Fuggle S, Taube D, Galliford J, Mamode N, Ball S, R Rommel, Torpey N, Bradley A. UK Registry of Antibody Incompatible Transplantation 2001–2009. 2010; Glasgow, UK: British Transplant Society Annual Congress.

67 Cosio FG, Gloor JM, Sethi S, Stegall MD. Transplant glomerulopathy. *American Journal of Transplantation* 2008;8(3):492–496.

68 Kobayashi T, Liu D, Ogawa H, Miwa Y, Nagasaka T, Maruyama S, *et al.* Removal of blood group A/B antigen in organs by ex vivo and in vivo administration of endo-beta-galactosidase (ABase) for ABO-incompatible transplantation. *Transplant Immunology* 2009;20(3):132–138.

69 Stegall MD, Diwan T, Raghavaiah S, Cornell LD, Burns J, Dean PG, *et al.* Terminal complement inhibition decreases antibody-mediated rejection in sensitized renal transplant recipients. *American Journal of Transplantation* 2011;11(11):2405–2413.

70 Perry DK, Burns JM, Pollinger HS, Amiot BP, Gloor JM, Gores GJ, *et al.* Proteasome inhibition causes apoptosis of normal human plasma cells preventing alloantibody production. *American Journal of Transplantation* 2009;9(1):201–209.

71 Trivedi HL, Terasaki PI, Feroz A, Everly MJ, Vanikar AV, Shankar V, *et al.* Abrogation of anti-HLA antibodies via proteasome inhibition. *Transplantation* 2009;87(10):1555–1561.

72 Sberro-Soussan R, Zuberl J, Suberbielle-Boissel C, Legendre C. Bortezomib alone fails to decrease donor specific anti-HLA antibodies: even after one year post-treatment. *Clinical Transplants* 2010:409–414.

5 Pancreas Transplantation

Rajinder Singh[1], David E.R. Sutherland[2], and Raja Kandaswamy[2]

[1]Guy's and St Thomas' Hospital, Great Ormond Street Hospital, UK
[2]Department of Surgery, University of Minnesota, USA

Introduction

Pancreas transplantation has become a more applicable option for treating insulin-dependent diabetes mellitus over the last 3 decades [1].

Type-1 diabetes mellitus has two treatments: (a) exogenous insulin administration or (b) β-cell replacement by pancreas or islet transplantation. The former is burdensome to the patient and gives imperfect glycemic control, predisposing to secondary complications of the eyes, nerves, kidneys, and other systems. The latter, when successful, establishes a constant euglycemic state but requires major surgery—at least for the pancreas transplant—and immunosuppression to prevent rejection, predisposing to complications as well, often compounded by those that are preexisting from diabetes.

Because of the established lack of sustained success with islet transplantation [2], solid-organ pancreas transplantation remains the gold standard for β-cell replacement. With refinement in surgical techniques, the availability of better immunosuppression, and lessons learned from previous experience, the results of pancreas transplantation have improved significantly [1,3–5]. This improvement has brought a paradigm shift in the current approach towards a patient with diabetes mellitus, in that the main aspects considered are the overall surgical/anesthetic candidacy and the benefit in trading off the need for insulin administration to that of immunosuppression.

Diabetes mellitus

According to the World Health Organization (WHO), the age-standardized worldwide adult diabetes prevalence in 2008 was 9.8% (range 8.6–11.2) in men and 9.2% (8.0–10.5) in women, which has gone up from 8.3% (6.5–10.4) and 7.5% (5.8–9.6) in 1980. The number of people with diabetes

Abdominal Organ Transplantation: State of the Art, First Edition.
Edited by Nizam Mamode and Raja Kandaswamy.
© 2013 Blackwell Publishing Ltd. Published 2013 by Blackwell Publishing Ltd.

increased from 153 (127–182) million in 1980 to 347 (314–382) million in 2008 [6]. This number is expected to touch 438 million by 2030. The current prevalence ranges from 10.2% in the Western Pacific to 3.8% in the African region, and diabetes is a leading cause of premature illness and death worldwide.

According to the American Diabetes Association [7], the prevalence of diabetes in Americans aged 60 or more is about 18.3%. Diabetic nephropathy accounts for 40% of newly diagnosed cases of end-stage renal disease in the USA. It is seen in 20–30% cases of type-1 or 2 diabetics, but a greater proportion of those with type 1 deteriorate to require dialysis. However, given the significantly larger number of type-2 diabetics in comparison to type-1, the former account for nearly half of the diabetics requiring dialysis. And among dialysis patients, those with diabetes have higher annual costs and mortality [8].

Diabetes management

Insulin versus pancreas transplantation

The requirement for insulin administration affects the quality of life of an individual. Not only is it a burden, but there is often suboptimal control of blood sugars, which can lead to the development of microvascular complications affecting the kidneys, eyes, and nerves, to name but a few. Studies have shown that intensive insulin therapy does improve, but rarely normalizes, glycosylated-hemoglobin levels and helps in the reduction of diabetic microvascular complications [4,9,10]. Perfect glycemic control is extremely difficult to achieve even with the most rigorous and meticulous insulin delivery options, and even if achieved, rates of secondary complications remain high [11,12]. On the other hand, it can be achieved through solid-organ pancreas transplantation, with normalization of glycosylated hemoglobin levels [13,14]. Pancreas transplantation can restore the production of endogenous insulin, and also help in the counterregulation of glucose metabolism. There is normalization of glucose metabolism at cellular and systemic level, and normalization of glucose homeostasis, translating into avoidance of hyperglycemia and hypoglycemia episodes [15,16]. With the patient rendered insulin-free through a successful pancreas transplant, there is also an improvement in quality of life, a reduction as well as reversal of some microvascular complications, and an elimination of the cumbersome process of daily insulin injections and frequent glucose monitoring. In the long term, it stabilizes retinopathy, improves neuropathy, causes regression of nephropathy by improving glomerular architecture, reverses interstitial expansion, resorps atrophic tubules, and improves macrovascular disease, cardiac function, and endothelial function [17–26]. These improvements occur in addition to the alleviation of anxiety relating to frequent administration of insulin. However, there is no improvement in advanced vascular disease and retinopathy [27]. Therefore, the advantages of transplanting a pancreas are greater if it is done before the onset of severe complications.

Pancreas transplantation versus islet-cell transplantation

Islet-cell transplantation, another type of β-cell replacement, is usually performed using deceased-donor pancreata. Current criteria in the USA preferentially allocate donors over age 50 and with body mass index (BMI) >30 to islet transplants. The process entails extraction of islet cells from the pancreas by enzymatic digestion of the parenchyma, and subsequent purification to obtain the islet-cell preparation. The islet cells are then injected into the portal vein of the recipient, usually by radiological or minimally invasive surgical techniques.

Interest in islet transplantation was revived in the late 1990s after the "Edmonton Protocol," using a steroid-free nondiabetogenic immunosuppression protocol [28] that showed high insulin-independence rates at 1 year post-transplant. Similar results from single-donor islet-cell transplants have been reported from the University of Minnesota, utilizing a similar regimen, but these included donors with a high BMI whose islets were transplanted to recipients with a lower BMI, thereby transplanting a similar net islet number per unit weight to that of the Alberta series [29].Currently, the success rates of insulin independence, although promising in the short term, tend to taper in the long term, with graft function—even after multiple-donor islet-cell transplants—about 10% at 5 years post-transplantation [30]. The suboptimal success rates have been attributed to a variety of causes [31], but the results are continuing to improve [2,32,33]. A recent Collaborative Islet Transplant Registry (CITR) report showed significantly improved islet-graft survival rates [2]. This study found that among 325 adult recipients of 649 islet infusions derived from 712 donors, at 3 years post-first infusion, 23% of islet-alone recipients were insulin-independent, 29% were insulin-dependent (but with detectable C-peptide), and 26% lost function. The remaining 22% had missing data. About 70% achieved insulin independence at least once, of whom 71% maintained status quo 1 year later and 52% at 2 years. However, the success rates were favored by higher numbers of infusions and of total islet equivalents infused, lower pretransplant glycosylated hemoglobin levels, processing centers related to the transplant center, and larger islet size. Use of protocols with daclizumab or etanercept during induction lowered the rates of function loss and achieved higher rates of insulin-independence.

Until islet transplants can consistently succeed from a single donor, regardless of recipient size or insulin requirements, an integrated approach is likely; large donors will be used for islet transplants to recipients with low insulin needs, and the remaining donors (the majority) for pancreas transplants to recipients with average or high insulin requirements. This strategy will maximize the number of recipients who receive allogeneic β-cells and eliminate surgical complications for at least a subset of patients.

Pancreas transplantation: a routine technique?

Around 35 000 pancreas transplants have been performed worldwide, of which 24 000 were performed in the USA (Figures 5.1 and 5.2). Currently,

Pancreas Transplants 12/16/1966 – 2009

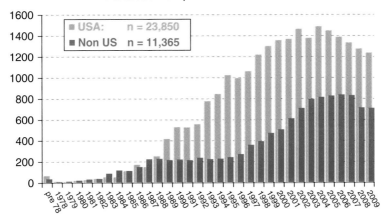

Figure 5.1 Pancreas transplants performed in the USA and worldwide. Reproduced with permission from Angelika Gruessner, International Registry of Pancreas Transplantation

USA Pancreas Transplants 1/1/1988 – 2010

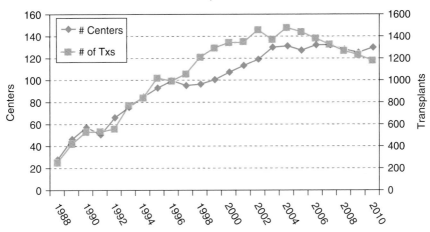

Figure 5.2 Number of transplant (Tx) centers and number of pancreas transplants in the USA. Reproduced with permission from Angelika Gruessner, International Registry of Pancreas Transplantation

about 1200 pancreas transplants are performed annually in the USA, and about 800 in the rest of the world. Of these, 75% are simultaneous pancreas–kidney (SPK) transplants, 18% are pancreas after kidney (PAK) transplants, and 7% are pancreas transplants alone (PTAs). Despite an initial increase in numbers, pancreas transplants have declined since 2004, with the largest decrease seen in the PAK category (by 50%), and a decline in SPKs of 7% from 2004 to 2010. An analysis of US pancreas transplantation over different eras showed that the mean recipient age at transplantation increased from 25–35 years in 1988 to about 40 years in 2010. There has also been an increase in pancreas implants into type-2 diabetics (currently 8% for SPK, 5% for PAK, and 1% for PTA). However, donor selection has become more stringent, with an increasing number of transplants using younger donors and trauma victims, and with shorter preservation time (mean 10–12 hours currently). There has been an increase in pancreas retransplants (currently 2% for SPK, 22% for PAK, and 18% for PTA), African-American recipients (currently 18% for SPK and 6% for PAK and PTA). Enteric drainage is currently the predominant duct-drainage technique (90% for SPK and PAK and 84% for PTA), and systemic venous drainage is the predominant venous drainage used (82% for SPK and PAK and 90% for PTA). Immunosuppressive protocols commonly use antibody induction with tacrolimus/mycophenolate mofetil as major maintenance therapy. Steroid avoidance has also increased in all three categories of pancreas transplant (30% for SPK and 48% for PAK and PTA).

Indications and contraindications for pancreas transplantation

The indication for pancreas transplantation differs for diabetic patients with normal renal function versus those with renal failure. For those with normal renal function, the foremost indication is hypoglycemia unawareness and labile diabetes with frequent insulin reactions. In diabetics whose autonomic nerves have been affected by longstanding hyperglycemia [34], episodes of hypoglycemia unawareness may occur, where the usual neural and cardiac warning signs of impending low sugars, such as restlessness, anxiety, and sense of impending death, are masked and they are unable to take remedial measures. This can potentially pose a threat to life (self or others) or cause irreversible brain damage. In those who have labile diabetes, the risks of a surgical procedure and consequences of immunosuppression may be preferable to the burden of a lifetime of diabetes [12,35]. Even among those without the above mentioned symptoms, many would prefer to have a pancreas transplant instead of carrying a lifetime burden of managing diabetes with insulin. In these candidates, however, it is unclear whether the long-term risks of diabetes are overcome by the risks of immunosuppression.

   In contrast, the uremic diabetic is frequently considered for pancreas transplantation, in addition to kidney [36]. The risks of immunosuppression are already assumed because of the need for a kidney transplant, so a simultaneous or sequential pancreas transplant does not pose significant additional risks, other than surgical ones. Traditionally, uremic individuals with type-1 diabetes are offered a pancreas along with a kidney [36]. Recent literature on transplantation of the pancreas in type-2 diabetics is also promising [37–39]. It has been noted that survival is poor in uremic diabetics [40,41], who have the highest rate of mortality on the waiting list for transplantation [8,42]. Therefore, in most circumstances, transplanting a pancreas along with a kidney is justified in uremic patients with insulin-dependent diabetes, whether type 1 or 2. In addition, a functioning pancreas transplant prevents recurrence of disease in a functioning kidney transplant in the long run, by providing a milieu of normoglycemia. It is worthwhile to note that according to the American Diabetes Association, 30–40% of patients with type-1 or 2 diabetes progress to end-stage renal disease, and that diabetic nephropathy is currently the most common cause of end-stage renal disease, accounting for about 40% of newly diagnosed patients. Given the significantly larger number of type-2 diabetics in comparison to type-1, the former account for nearly half of diabetics requiring dialysis [8].

The recipient selection criteria for pancreas-transplant patients aged 18–65 years are an ability to withstand surgery and immunosuppression, psychosocial stability, social support, compliance and a commitment to long-term follow-up, the presence of secondary complications of diabetes or hyperlability ("complicated diabetes"), and the absence of any exclusion criteria. The exclusion criteria include insufficient cardiovascular reserve, coronary angiographic evidence of uncorrectable coronary artery disease or ejection fraction below 30%, recent myocardial infarction, ongoing substance abuse (drug or alcohol), major ongoing psychiatric illness, recent noncompliance, lack of social support, active infection or recent malignancy, lack of well-defined diabetic complications, and significant obesity (BMI $>30–35\,kg/m^2$).

Renal replacement therapy in diabetics

Studies have shown that there is a survival benefit for SPK versus deceased- (and possibly living-) donor kidney transplant alone, and for SPK and PAK transplants (and possibly PTA) verus remaining on the waiting list [43–47]. In selected diabetic patients, adding a simultaneous pancreas to a kidney transplant results in improvement of the results of pancreas transplantation and does not adversely affect either patient or kidney graft survival. Apart from being an acutely life-enhancing modality, SPK transplant is also life-prolonging.

Expansion of the donor pool

Due to a continued organ shortage and an increase in diabetics as well as in diabetic nephropathy, continued inroads are being made into increasing the existing donor pool. The main areas have been the use of donation after cardiac death (or DCD), the use of older donors, and the use of segmental grafts from living donors.

DCD donors

There has been a significant increase in the number of pancreata transplanted from DCD (or asystolic) donors over the last few years [5,38,48–51]. The reported outcomes from these donors have been shown to be excellent, but more stringent criteria are imposed on them to ensure that they are relatively younger and have no other significant comorbidity, and that the cold-ischemia times are lower [50]. Recently, some authors have reported the use of extracorporeal interval support for organ retrieval (EISOR) for renal and extra-renal organ procurement [38]. Despite having small numbers in the study group, they have shown 100% patient and pancreas graft survival, at least on short-term follow-up, as well as rates of delayed graft function in the kidneys significantly lower than those seen in kidneys transplanted from conventional DCD donors. The process entails pre-mortem cannulae placement, with the consent of donor family members, prior to withdrawal of life support. After declaration of death, and a requisite wait of 5 minutes of cardiac arrest, the organs are perfused by starting cold perfusion, and the procurement is performed in a controlled fashion. However, potential problems of cardiac reanimation and ongoing cerebral flow with EISOR may be an issue, and this process has not yet gained widespread acceptance, given the ethical and sensitivity issues involved. In another study [38], the authors compared the outcomes of an extended donor-criteria pancreas transplant cohort of SPKs (which were defined as age $\geq$ 45 years or DCD) with SPKs from conventional donors, and given a similar median follow-up of 29 months, patient, kidney, and pancreatic graft survival rates, delayed graft-function rates, rejections and infections, and surgical complication rates were similar. The 1-year mean serum creatinine or glycohemoglobin were also similar between the two groups.

Solid-organ pancreas transplants from living donors

Pancreas transplants have been performed in the past using living donors (Figure 5.3) and the long-term graft survival rate is reported to be significantly higher for living- (versus deceased-) donor pancreas transplant recipients [52]. The first living-donor segmental pancreas transplant was done at the University of Minnesota in 1979, and insulin-independence was achieved [53–56]. There have since been more than 150 cases reported worldwide (124 reported from the University of Minnesota) [57]. In the Minnesota experience [55,57,58], the reason for choosing a living donor, initially for solitary pancreas transplants (PAK, PTA), was due to the high

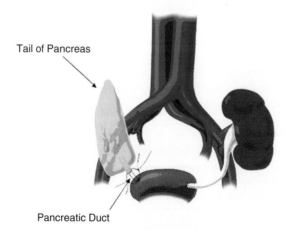

Tail of Pancreas

Pancreatic Duct

Figure 5.3 Simultaneous pancreas (segmental) kidney transplantation from a living donor

rejection and low survival rates seen with pancreata from deceased-donor grafts, along with a shortage of deceased-donor grafts. The complications reported in the recipients of living-donor SPKs included thrombosis in 3%, pancreatic enzyme leak in 5%, bleeding in 4%, abscess formation in 7%, and infected aneurysm in 1%. The pancreas technical failure rate was 11% and the postoperative mortality was nil. The incidence of development of diabetes in the donors by formal studies was about 30%, and 6% were on insulin. However, with the application of stricter preselection criteria, the insulin-dependent diabetes risk in the donor was reduced to 1%.

Potential donors may undergo either segmental pancreas donation alone (for non-uremic or post-uremic recipients) or simultaneous segmental pancreas and unilateral kidney donation (for uremic recipients). Once identified, potential donors should be subjected to a thorough medical, metabolic, and psychosocial screening. ABO and human leukocyte antigen (HLA) cross-match compatibility is preferred but not mandatory. A segmental donor pancreatectomy can also be applied for islet isolation and allotransplantation, if facilities for islet-cell isolation are available.

Expansion of the recipient pool

An International Pancreas Transplant Registry (IPTR) analysis [1,5] shows that there has been an increase in pancreas transplants implanted into diabetic uremic recipients with measureable C peptide (or type-2 diabetics), older donors, African-American ethnicity, pancreatic retransplants, major HLA locus mismatch, and HLA sensitization.

Transplanting type-2 diabetics

There has been a paradigm shift in the approach towards selecting diabetic uremic candidates for transplantation. Traditional criteria for accepting recipients for pancreas transplantation required type-1 diabetics [59]. Transplantation in patients who are C-peptide positive, or who are type-2 diabetics, is a topic of ongoing discussion. Individuals belonging to this subset are usually older, obese, of African descent, and have peripheral insulin resistance. But the common thought that they cannot benefit from a pancreas transplant has been challenged by several studies, and currently most of the available evidence suggests that they do indeed benefit and become insulin-independent [37,39,60]. A study done in the University of Minnesota [60] showed that pancreas transplants can provide excellent glucose control in recipients with type-2 diabetes. All 16 of their recipients whose transplant was technically successful (94%) were rendered euglycemic. Long-term results were comparable with those seen in transplant recipients with type-1 diabetes. A study from Wake Forest University [37] compared outcomes between patients with absent or low pretransplant C-peptide levels (2.0 ng/ml) and those with levels of 2.0 ng/ml who received an SPK transplant, and given a similar median follow-up of 40 months the death-censored kidney and pancreas graft survival rates were similar, but patient survival was slightly lower in the C-peptide-positive recipients. The latter were older, showed a later age of onset of diabetes, weighed more, included a greater proportion of African-Americans, and had a longer pretransplant duration of dialysis. It is speculated that the increase in β-cell mass helps overcome insulin resistance or challenges the theory of insulin resistance. However, it has to be taken into account that the procedural and postoperative complications could be higher in these individuals due to their obesity and cardiac status. It has also been observed that they have continued need for oral hypoglycemic agents, despite being insulin-free [37].

Currently approved organ allocation policy in the USA (pending implementation) allows allocation of kidney–pancreata and pancreata to insulin-dependent, non-obese, C-peptide-positive recipients.

Therefore, to summarize, the current evidence suggests that the main consideration for SPK and PAK is the surgical risk, and the main consideration for PTA is hypoglycemia unawareness. There is little reason not to do an SPK or PAK transplant in non-obese insulin-dependent type-2 diabetics. PTA is largely limited to hypoglycemia unawareness and nearly all patients are C-peptide-negative. If a true hypoglycemia-unaware C-peptide-positive PTA candidate exists, the transplant should be done. The C peptide is of importance only in that hypoglycemia unawareness is rare if positive.

Recipient pretransplant work-up

Pretransplant work-up should include a detailed history, cardiopulmonary risk assessment, and vascular examination. Most transplant candidates may require coronary angiograms, since noninvasive tests such as myoview scan are not good predictors of cardiac risk in long-standing diabetes [61,62]. In healthy young subjects, dobutamine stress echocardiograms may suffice [63]. If coronary artery disease is detected on angiograms, angioplasty/stenting or surgical revascularization is indicated, and such patients have a lower rate of postoperative cardiac complications compared to those with medical therapy alone [64]. Assessment of the iliac vasculature is important, usually using a duplex scan.

Choice of operation: SPK/PAK/PTA

The three common types of operation performed for pancreas transplant are SPK, PAK, and PTA. These techniques have been described and evolved based on experience [65–69]. According to the latest IPTR report [5], of the 35 000 pancreas transplants performed worldwide that were reported, 75% were SPK, 18% were PAK, and 7% were PTA. Pancreas transplantation usually involves placement of the pancreas intraperitoneally, although some centers are implanting in an extraperitoneal position[69]. PTA is performed for hypogycaemia unawareness, as described earlier.

For uremic diabetics, both a kidney and a pancreas are transplanted, and this can be done either as an SPK or as a PAK transplantation. Which is performed usually depends on the availability of pancreas and kidney donors. Because survival of uremic diabetics is poor on the waiting list, it may be prudent to transplant a kidney from a living donor as soon as one is available. The kidney recipient can then go on to receive a pancreas transplantation from a deceased donor whenever a suitable one becomes available. This is known as PAK. In this scenario, two separate operations are required. The kidney transplant is usually implanted into the left iliac fossa, and the right side is reserved for the future pancreas transplant. The iliac vessels, especially the veins, are more superficial on the right side, and therefore this side is preferentially preserved for pancreas transplantation, which is technically the more challenging of the two operations. Moreover, the portal vein in the pancreas allograft is considerably shorter in length than the renal vein, and it is technically easier to suture this into the right side than the left side. Those who do not have a living donor must remain on the waiting list for both kidney and pancreas from a deceased donor. In some circumstances, a living-donor kidney can be timed with deceased-donor pancreas transplantation, if the living donor is available to come for donation at short notice.

SPK and PTA have also been performed from living donors. For an SPK, where the donor has consented to donate a pancreas as well as a kidney, a segment of pancreas is removed simultaneously with the kidney. This is most commonly done in conjunction with a left-donor nephrectomy, as the distal pancreas is located in the vicinity. In the past, the process of removal of kidney and pancreas was done by the open technique, but currently the laparoscopic technique is used. The process of removal of pancreas increases both surgical morbidity and the risk of developing diabetes in the future. However, the frequency of such adverse events has significantly declined, due to the application of stringent donor-selection criteria and refinement in surgical techniques.

Surgical aspects of pancreas transplantation

Pancreas transplantation surgery comprises back-table benchwork preparation of the pancreas (and kidneys, for SPK), dissection of the blood vessels for implantation, and implantation of the organs.

Back-table benchwork

Before proceeding with transplantation, it is essential for the implanting surgeon to visualize the pancreas and the kidney, in order to ensure that the organs are appropriate for transplantation. It is not uncommon to see that the pancreas has suffered injury during retrieval, or that it is of poor quality. Along with the pancreas, the donor "Y" graft is also inspected, to ensure that there is no injury at its "crotch." Usually, the left kidney is preferred over the right, due to the longer renal vein—if the right kidney is used, a venous extension may be employed to ensure that implantation of the renal vein is facilitated.

Surgical technique of implantation

The implantation of a pancreas into the recipient requires three anastomoses to be created. These are: venous anastomosis for outflow; arterial anastomosis for inflow; and exocrine drainage. During an SPK transplant, the pancreas transplant is usually performed first, because this organ is more adversely affected by an increase in the cold-ischemia time. The pancreas is implanted into the right iliac fossa, and the kidney into the left iliac fossa. Occasionally, some surgeons may prefer to do the kidney implantation first, if the cold time is short. The reason for doing this is that repositioning of the retractor blades is avoided. If a pancreas is implanted first, the retractors have to be repositioned to expose the left side for the kidney anastomoses, and this maneuver can potentially jeopardize the implanted pancreas allograft directly, or else adversely affect the anastomosis.

Venous drainage: portal versus systemic drainage

The most common form of venous drainage (using the pancreatic portal vein) is systemic (Figures 5.4 and 5.5), usually to the right common iliac vein. Depending on the recipient anatomy and body habitus, the right

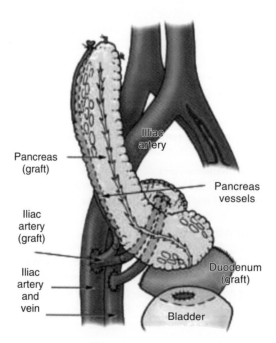

Figure 5.4 Systemic bladder drainage technique of pancreas transplantation

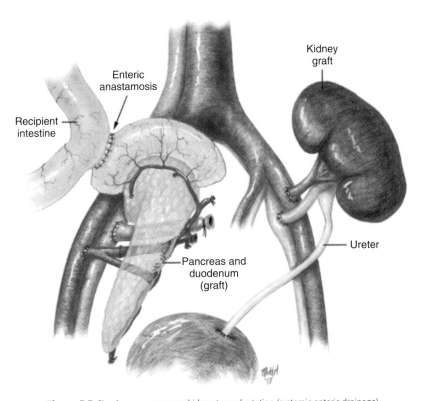

Kidney
graft

Enteric
anastamosis

Recipient
intestine

Ureter

Pancreas and
duodenum
(graft)

Figure 5.5 Simultaneous pancreas kidney transplantation (systemic enteric drainage)

external iliac vein or even the inferior vena cava (IVC) may also be used. Mobilization of the iliac veins usually requires division of the internal iliac veins. When the iliac veins are used, the pancreas is usually positioned "head down," meaning that the donor pancreas with its "C" loop of duodenum in positioned facing inferiorly. This makes it possible for the donor duodenum to be anastomosed either to the recipient urinary bladder or to the recipient small bowel, whichever is chosen. If the IVC is used for the portal venous anastomosis, the pancreas has to be positioned "head up," and it would be difficult in this situation to do a bladder exocrine drainage. Exocrine drainage is usually performed enterically in this situation. One of the reasons for using the IVC for anastomosis is that this obviates the need for extensive dissection and mobilization of the iliac veins, which can be technically challenging.

Some centers [66,70–72] have advocated for the use of a recipient portal venous system for venous drainage (Figure 5.6). The donor pancreas portal vein is anastomosed to the recipient superior mesenteric vein (or its major radical), and less frequently the splenic vein (Figure 5.6). The argument in favor of this technique is that this is more physiological. The insulin produced by the transplant pancreas will not enter the systemic circulation directly (which might increase the risk of hyperinsulinemia), but rather

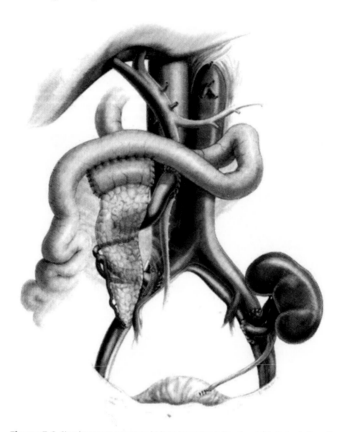

Figure 5.6 Simultaneous pancreas kidney transplantation (portal enteric drainage)

through the liver undergoing first-pass metabolism, mimicking the normal physiological situation. Some authors [66] have shown portal venous drainage to be associated with lower graft-rejection rates, but there has been no real evidence favoring one technique over the other [5,71,73]. When using portal venous drainage, exocrine drainage will have to be enteric, since the position of the pancreas makes it impossible to anastomose the duodenum to the bladder. IPTR data in 2005 showed that among exocrine-drainage transplants, venous drainage via the portal system was used for 20% of SPK, 23% of PAK, and 35% of PTA cases [73].

Arterial anastomosis

This is normally performed using a Y graft, derived from the donor common, external, and internal iliac arteries. The donor superior mesenteric and splenic arteries are each anastomosed to either limb of the Y graft, and the main stem of the graft is then anastomosed to the recipient common iliac artery or aorta.

With portal venous drainage, the common stem of the Y graft is brought through a small opening in the root of the mesentery and anastomosed to the recipient right common iliac artery. Quite often, an extension graft has to be attached to the common Y stem to provide enough length to reach the iliacs when using this technique of venous drainage.

Exocrine drainage: bladder versus enteric drainage

Solid-organ pancreas transplantation provides both endocrine and exocrine function. The latter is unnecessary, but exocrine drainage is an unavoidable part of the procedure and is responsible for many of the postoperative complications. Drainage is into either the recipient urinary bladder (Figure 5.4) or the recipient small bowel (Figures 5.5 and 5.6). Duct injections have also been used in the past, in an attempt to obliterate the exocrine system [74,75]. In the current era, the pancreas allograft is procured, along with the "C" loop of duodenum around it. This duodenal segment collects the allograft exocrine juices and delivers them to either the bladder or the bowel. Both methods have their advantages and disadvantages. Bladder drainage is nonphysiological and has side effects such as pancreatitis, dehydration, urinary complications, and urinary-tract infections, to name a few. In about 10%, the symptoms are severe enough to justify converting them to bowel drainage at some point in the future; this process is called "enteric conversion." The advantages of bladder drainage include assessment of urinary amylase, a reduction in which may be an early pointer for pancreas allograft rejection. Usually, when a pancreas allograft is lost through rejection, the exocrine part is affected before the endocrine part. Therefore, hyperglycemia is a late marker for pancreas rejection. Transcystoscopic pancreas biopsies are also possible with this technique. Enteric drainage, on the other hand, is physiological, and does not have the usual side effects of bladder drainage. It does however have its own set of adverse complications, such as enteric leak, sepsis, and bowel obstruction. Furthermore, rejection cannot be monitored with urinary amylase, and no opportunity exists for transcystoscopic biopsies. The usual recourse is to monitor the serum amylase and lipase as indirect markers of pancreas rejection, with a computed tomography (CT)-guided transabdominal pancreas biopsy for confirmation. Such biopsies do, however, carry significant risks, including bleeding and allograft loss.

Postoperative management

Initial care after pancreas transplantation is similar to care after any major surgical procedure. Surgical intensive-care unit (ICU) for 24–48 hours is recommended, and assessment is 1–2-hourly. Monitoring of graft function by glucose levels is mandatory. Any sudden unexplained increase in glucose levels, especially >11 mmol/l, should raise suspicion of graft thrombosis, and urgent Doppler evaluation of the pancreas transplant should be undertaken to assess blood flow to the graft. In case of persisting doubt, the patient should be returned to theater for reexploration. Tight glycemic control (<8 mmol/l) with an intravenous (IV) insulin drip is used by some to "rest" the pancreas in the early postoperative period. Elevation of serum amylase or lipase may suggest graft pancreatitis or acute rejection. If a drain is left in, measurement of amylase in the drain effluent is performed, and persistent elevation and increased output maybe due to pancreatic exocrine leakage or graft pancreatitis. Use of low-dose heparin in the early postoperative period (days 0–5) reduces the risk of graft thrombosis [76], especially for PTA. Enteric coated aspirin 81 mg is started on postoperative day 1 and continued for 6 months. Use of an octeotide infusion may help to reduce the incidence of complications in pancreas transplant recipients [77], and may also be indicated during persistent leakage of pancreas enzymes in the drains. Being a "low-flow" organ, intravascular volume must be maintained to provide adequate perfusion to the pancreas allograft. Dehydration and metabolic acidosis are more frequently associated with bladder-drained pancreas transplantation. A bladder catheter is usually kept for 5–10 days, and after its removal a post-void ultrasound scan is recommended to ensure adequate drainage of the urinary bladder, given the incidence of autonomic neuropathy in diabetic patients. Broad-based antibiotic therapy (with strong Gram-negative coverage and antifungal therapy) is instituted in the operating room prior to incision, and continued for 3–7 days. Antiviral prophylaxis, for cytomegalovirus (CMV) for example, is similar to that in other solid-organ transplants.

Immunosuppression

Along with improvements in surgical technique and postoperative care, the success of pancreas transplantation over the last few decades has also been attributed to better immunosuppressive regimens [5]. Azathioprine and prednisolone used to be the mainstays of immunosuppression, until the advent of cyclosporine in the mid 1980s [78]. Cyclosporine made a significant impact on the survival of allograft, with a reduction in rejection rates [78,79]. Subsequently, in the mid 1990s, tacrolimus and mycophenolate mofetil were introduced into the transplant arena, and they have become the major maintenance immunosuppressive agents in pancreas transplantation, with significantly better outcomes over cyclosporine-based regimes [79–81]. With the recent introduction of anti-T-cell antibody induction (depleting and nondepleting, polyvalent and monovalent), the rejection rates have continued to improve. The T-cell-depleting antibodies include rabbit antithymocyte globulin (rATG) (polyvalent) and alemtuzumab (anti-CD53, monovalent), and the nondepleting antibodies include basiliximab and daclizumab (IL-2 R antagonists). Currently about 88% of pancreas transplant recipients receive antibody induction therapy and 65% receive tacrolimus/mycophenolate mofetil maintenance, with successful steroid elimination in 40–50%. There has been a trend towards increased usage of depleting antibodies, and a decline in usage of nondepleting antibodies [82]. The results of alemtuzumab induction appear quite promising, and a random controlled trial comparing this with rATG, with tacrolimus/mycophenolate mofetil maintenance, has shown significantly lower pancreas allograft rejection rates in the alemtuzumab group [83].

T-cell-depleting antibodies provide an umbrella of protection, which has encouraged attempts at steroid elimination, calcineurin-inhibitor (CNI) minimization/elimination, and tacrolimus monotherapy, in the hope of improving long-term outcomes [84–89]. Steroid elimination has been possible in pancreas transplantation, using both alemtuzumab and rATG induction, with low rates of rejection. However, CNI avoidance/minimization has been less promising, at least so far. Tacrolimus monotherapy with alemtuzumab induction has been successfully attempted, with good results, in short-term follow-up studies. Further studies are needed however before the role of tacrolimus monotherapy is definitely established. Immune monitoring has been used to guide immunosuppression recently. The ImmuKnow Assay (Cylex Inc., Columbia, MD) has been used to aid immunosuppression in pancreas transplantation by comparing the T-cell responses in various clinical states [90]. An assay of <100 ATP ng/ml correlated with over-immunosuppression and infection, whereas an assay of >500 ATP ng/ml correlated with underimmunosuppression and rejection. The authors recommend aiming for a level of 200 ATP ng/ml on the ImmuKnow Assay, since this correlated with optimal immunosuppression. Similarly, immune monitoring with Cylex, as well as flow-panel reactive antibody, has been used to guide rATG induction with sirolimus maintenance therapy in order to allow steroid elimination and CNI minimization/withdrawal in recipients showing a reduced immune response [91].

Outcomes

Outcomes are based on the United Network for Organ Sharing (UNOS)/ IPTR analysis as reported in various publications [1,5,73,92–94].

Patient and graft survival
According to the IPTR/UNOS registry analysis, the 1-year patient survival is 95% for SPK (green) and PAK (red), and 97% for PTA (yellow) (Figure 5.7).

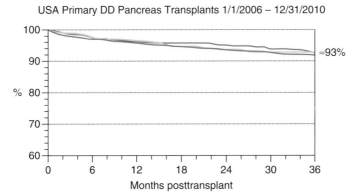

Figure 5.7 Patient survival in pancreas-transplant categories. Reproduced with permission from Angelika Gruessner, International Registry of Pancreas Transplantation

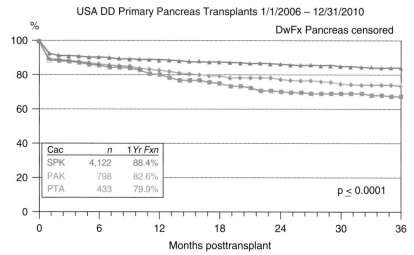

Figure 5.8 Pancreas survival in pancreas-transplant categories. Reproduced with permission from Angelika Gruessner, International Registry of Pancreas Transplantation

At 5 years, patient survival rates are 87% for SPK, 83% for PAK, and 87% for PTA transplants, and at 10 years the rates are 82%, 69%, and 72%, respectively. These figures have improved since 1988, when the respective survival rates were 78% for SPK and 66% for PAK/PTA transplants.

At 1-year post-transplant, death-censored pancreas survival is 88% for SPKs, 83% for PAK, and 80% for PTA (Figure 5.8). At 5 years, graft survival rates are 70%, 60%, and 52%, respectively. These figures have improved since 1988, when they were 60%, 20%, and 23%, respectively.

For the SPK patients, the 1-year kidney survival is 93%, and 5-year survival is 80%. This survival rate has improved from 68% in 1988.

The current 1-year immunological graft-loss rates are 1.8% for SPK, 3.7% for PAK, and 6% for PTA transplants. There has been a reduction in the 5-year immunological graft-loss rates, from 11% in 1988 to 9% in 2001 for SPK; from 65% in 1988 to 20% in 2001 for PAK; and from 75% in 1988 to 30% in 2001 for PTA.

At 2 years post-transplant, the pancreas graft loss from chronic rejection is 1.5% for SPK, 5.7% for PAK, and 10.3% for PTA.

There has also been a significant improvement in the early technical failure rate, which is currently down to 8–9%. For the PTAs, the technical complication rate is down from 25% in 1988 to 9% in 2006. For the SPKs/PAKs, the technical complication rate is down from 11% in 1988 to 9% in 2006.

Surgical complications

Technically, pancreas transplantation is a very demanding procedure, and meticulous attention to detail is paramount for a reduction in the complication rates. However, despite best efforts, complications are not infrequent, and mainly include graft thrombosis, bleeding, abdominal-fluid collections, and infections.

Graft thrombosis

With improvements in surgical technique, graft thrombosis rates have declined. Thrombosis is seen either in the pancreas portal venous anastomosis or in the Y arterial graft. The main causes are usually technical, hypotension in the postoperative period, or poor graft quality. A sudden surge in the insulin requirement should prompt radiological investigations (usually a Doppler flow study of the graft,). The reported incidence of pancreas-graft thrombosis is 5–13% [76,95]. Short portal veins requiring extension grafts, a segmental pancreas allograft, atherosclerotic arteries in the donor or recipient, narrow pelvic inlet with deeply placed iliac vein, a technically difficult anastomosis, kinks in the vessels, hypercoagulable states such as factor-V Leiden mutation, presence of lupus anticoagulant, deficiencies of antithrombin, protein-C or S or activated protein-C resistance are some of the causes of this serious complication[96–98]. If it is detected late, it invariably necessitates graft pancreatectomy.

For SPK transplants, the kidney allografts are also at risk of developing thrombosis. Again, technical reasons, as well as some of the other reasons cited here, predominate. In addition, torsion of the renal pedicle has also been reported [99,100]. Given the intraperitoneal location of the kidney, it is more mobile, and long pedicles (>5 cm) can predispose to torsion. Renopexy is one recommended way of preventing this complication.

Postoperative bleeding

This is a common cause of immediate return to theater, and the reported incidence is 6–8% [95,101]. Use of heparin in the perioperative period may predispose to development of this complication. A reexploration is required if the bleeding does not settle despite cessation of heparin, correction of coagulation parameters if abnormal, or if there is massive bleeding as evident from the drain output, hemodynamic instability, or deranged hematological parameters. Sometimes, bleeding can arise from the graft duodenum [102] early in the postoperative period. The causes include bleeding from the anastomotic suture lines, a raw area of duodenum, and acute rejection manifested in the duodenal component of the pancreatico-duodenal allograft. This may necessitate graft pancreatectomy [103] if conservative management such as octreotide infusion or treatment of the cause (if known) fails to ameliorate the situation.

Abdominal collections

These are a significant cause of morbidity and resource utilization, and may require multiple laparotomies and graft pancreatectomy. The major causes of abdominal-fluid collections are pancreatic enzyme leaks from the duodenal stump or the pancreatic parenchyma, graft pancreatitis, acute rejection, and abdominal infection. The incidence of duodenal leak is reported to range from 4 to 6% [95,101], and it usually requires reexploration. Graft pancreatectomy may be required if there is gross abdominal contamination consequent to the leak. In less serious cases, a Roux-en-Y conversion may help, and in selected cases it may be used as a routine technique if there is any concern about the duodenal vascularity, in order to minimize the consequences of a leak. In some cases, a venting Roux-en-Y jejunostomy has been done [104]. If a duodenal stump leak occurs in bladder exocrine-drained pancreas transplants, it can usually be managed conservatively by prolonged decompression of the urinary bladder using a Foley catheter. Larger leaks may require surgical repair or an enteric conversion [105]. Relaparotomy and washouts are required for gross collections, multiple collections, or if there is no safe window for the radiologist to site the drain into a collection. Infected collections almost always require drainage, and surgical drainage maybe required in 4–10% of cases [95,101]. Intraoperative contamination during enteric anastomosis may predispose to abdominal infections. Gram-negative bacterial and fungal infections usually predominate. Some recipients may need multiple interventional radiological guided drainages or relaparotomies, can have sepsis, and quite often may have a persistent source of infection or enzyme leak. Such cases usually require graft pancreatectomy.

Other complications

These include wound infection, fascial dehiscence, hemorrhagic pancreatitis, pseudoaneurysms, severe rejection, and formation of arteriovenous fistula in the allograft.

Nonsurgical complications

The important nonsurgical complications include graft pancreatitis, acute rejection, and infectious complications. Less common, but still important, are graft-versus-host disease and post-transplant malignancies, especially lymphoproliferative diseases.

Bladder-drained pancreas transplants have a higher rate of graft pancreatitis than enteric-drained pancreas transplants. Urinary retention or incomplete bladder emptying may lead to an increased risk of these complications. The other causes of graft pancreatitis include immunosuppressive agents such as corticosteroids, azathioprine and cyclosporine, viral infections—especially cytomegalovirus and hepatitis C—hypercalcemia, and ischemia reperfusion injury. The diagnosis is usually based on a rise in serum amylase and lipase. Clinical manifestations such as tenderness over the graft and fever may or may not be present. For a bladder-drained pancreas, the management is by prolonged Foley catheterization and treatment of the underlying urologic cause. Repeated episodes may benefit from an enteric conversion [106–108]. Raised markers of pancreatic inflammation, such as serum amylase and lipase, may also be seen in graft rejection. It is often difficult to predict whether "graft pancreatitis" is from acute rejection or another cause. For bladder-drained pancreas transplants, serial measurement of urinary amylase showing a sustained decline from the baseline may indicate graft rejection, and a pancreas biopsy is indicated for confirmation [109]. In enteric-drained pancreas transplants, this tool of assessment is unavailable, and there is a major reliance on serum amylase or lipase as early markers of rejection [110]. Often, this leads to a pancreas allograft biopsy for confirmation [111,112]. Hyperglycemia due to rejection is usually a late event.

Risk factors for pancreas graft loss

The major risk factors for pancreas graft loss include donor factors such as age, BMI, prolonged intensive-care hospitalization (>48 hours) with a need for intensive vasoconstrictors, and prolonged hemodynamic instability, and recipient factors such as BMI and quality of blood vessels.

An elaborate analysis [113] of pancreas transplants has shown that SPK transplants have a slightly higher technical failure rate that PAK or PTA transplants (15% vs 12%). The same study showed that technical failure was the most important cause of pancreas graft loss. Thrombosis was seen to be the most important risk factor for technical failure (52%). Multivariate analysis showed recipient BMI >30, cold-ischemia time >12 hours, donor death from causes other than trauma, enteric versus bladder drainage, and donor BMI >30 to be the significant risk factors for technical failure. In this study, neither donor/recipient age nor retransplant was a risk factor for graft technical failure.

However, a vast majority of studies have shown donor age (especially >45 years) to be the most significant risk factor for pancreas graft loss [107,114–116].

The future

Avoidance of a major operation and achievement of glycemic control without exogenous insulin administration are the future goal. β-cell replacement can be derived from islet-cell transplants (deceased- or living-donor human islet allografts or xenografts), but these areas are still in development. Xenotransplantation has the major limitation of being affected by graft hyperacute rejection, and attempts are being made to avoid this by using an encapsulation technique [117–119]. This technique is also used for human islets, to minimize rejection episodes. However, human islet cells have less consistent results and poorer long-term survival, but do hold a promise for the future. Some are trying to generate islet cells from stem cells [120], but these projects are still in their infancy [121,122].

Therefore, at the current time, since solid-organ pancreas transplantation is the gold standard, studies are concentrating on further improving success rates by focusing on long-term graft survival in addition to short-term survival. These include using or trying to discover newer immunosuppressive regimens that are less nephrotoxic, avoiding steroids, minimizing or withdrawing use of CNIs, liberally using antibody induction agents, and trying to develop graft tolerance.

References

1 Gruessner AC, Sutherland DE. Pancreas transplant outcomes for United States (US) cases as reported to the United Network for Organ Sharing (UNOS) and the International Pancreas Transplant Registry (IPTR). *Clin Transpl* 2008:45–56.

2 Alejandro R, *et al.* Update from the Collaborative Islet Transplant Registry. *Transplantation* 2008;86(12):1783–8.

3 Burke GW, Ciancio G, Sollinger HW. Advances in pancreas transplantation. *Transplantation* 2004;77(9 Suppl):S62–67.

4 DCCT Research Group. Lifetime benefits and costs of intensive therapy as practiced in the diabetes control and complications trial. The Diabetes Control and Complications Trial Research Group. *JAMA* 1997(277).

5 Gruessner AC. 2011 update on pancreas transplantation: comprehensive trend analysis of 25,000 cases followed up over the course of twenty-four years at the International Pancreas Transplant Registry (IPTR). *Rev Diabet Stud* 2011;8(1):6–16.

6 Danaei G, Lin J, Farzadfar F, *et al*. National, regional, and global trends in fasting plasma glucose and diabetes prevalence since 1980: systematic analysis of health examination surveys and epidemiological studies with 370 country-years and 2·7 million participants. *The Lancet* 2001;378(9785):31–40.

7 dLife. Seniors and diabetes. 2007. http://www.dlife.com/diabetes/lifestyle /diabetes-seniors.

8 American Diabetic Association. Nephropathy in diabetes. *Diabetes Care* 2004;27(Suppl 1):S79–583.

9 The Diabetes Control and Complications Trial Research Group. The effect of intensive treatment of diabetes on the development and progression of long-term complications in insulin-dependent diabetes mellitus. *N Engl J Med* 1993;329(14):977–986.

10 DPT-1 Study Group. The Diabetes Prevention Trial—type 1 diabetes (DPT-1): implementation of screening and staging of relatives. *Transplant Proc* 1995;27(6):3377.

11 Krolewski AS, Warram JH, Freire MB. Epidemiology of late diabetic complications. A basis for the development and evaluation of preventive programs. *Endocrinol Metab Clin North Am* 1996;25(2):217–242.

12 Syndman DR. Infection in solid organ transplantation. *Transplant Infect Dis* 1999;1:21.

13 Morel P, *et al*. Long-term glucose control in patients with pancreatic transplants. *Ann Intern Med* 1991;115(9):694–699.

14 Morel P, *et al*. Serial glycosylated hemoglobin levels in diabetic recipients of pancreatic transplants. *Transplant Proc* 1990;22(2):649–650.

15 Robertson RP, Sutherland DE, Lanz KJ. Normoglycemia and preserved insulin secretory reserve in diabetic patients 10–18 years after pancreas transplantation. *Diabetes* 1999;48(9):1737–1740.

16 Paty BW, *et al*. Restored hypoglycemic counterregulation is stable in successful pancreas transplant recipients for up to 19 years after transplantation. *Transplantation* 2001;72(6):1103–1107.

17 Gruessner RW, *et al*. Simultaneous pancreas-kidney transplantation from live donors. *Ann Surg* 1997;226(4):471–480, disc. 480–482.

18 Sutherland D, Groth C. The history of pancreas transplantation. In: Hakim N, Papalois VE (eds) *History of Organ and Cell Transplantation*. 2003; London: Imperial College Press.

19 Kennedy WR, *et al*. Effects of pancreatic transplantation on diabetic neuropathy. *N Engl J Med* 1990;322(15):1031–1037.

20 Sutherland DE, *et al*. Pancreas transplantation in nonuremic, type I diabetic recipients. *Surgery* 1988;104(2):453–464.

21 van der Vliet JA, *et al*. The effect of pancreas transplantation on diabetic polyneuropathy. *Transplantation* 1988;45(2):368–370.

22 van der Vliet JA, *et al.* Diabetic polyneuropathy and renal transplantation. *Transplant Proc* 1987;19(5):3597–3599.

23 Solders G, *et al.* Improvement in nerve conduction 8 years after combined pancreatic and renal transplantation. *Transplant Proc* 1995;27(6):3091.

24 Solders G, *et al.* Improvement of nerve conduction in diabetic neuropathy. A follow-up study 4 yr after combined pancreatic and renal transplantation. *Diabetes* 1992;41(8):946–951.

25 Fioretto P, *et al.* Remodeling of renal interstitial and tubular lesions in pancreas transplant recipients. *Kidney Int* 2006;69(5):907–912.

26 Fiorina P, *et al.* Effects of kidney-pancreas transplantation on atherosclerotic risk factors and endothelial function in patients with uremia and type 1 diabetes. *Diabetes* 2001;50(3):496–501.

27 Stratta R. Impact of pancreas transplantation on complications of diabetes. *Curr Opin Organ Transplant* 1998;3:258.

28 Shapiro AM, *et al.* Islet transplantation in seven patients with type 1 diabetes mellitus using a glucocorticoid-free immunosuppressive regimen. *N Engl J Med*, 2000. 343(4):230–8.

29 Hering B, *et al.* Insulin independence after single donor islet transplantation in type-1 diabetes with hOKT-3-1 (ala-ala), sirolimus and tacrolimus therapy. *Am J Transplant* 2001;1:180.

30 Ryan EA, *et al.* Five-year follow-up after clinical islet transplantation. *Diabetes* 2005;54(7):2060–2069.

31 Hering B, Ricordi C. Islet transplantation for patients with type-1 diabetes. *Graft* 1999;2(12).

32 Matsumoto S. Islet cell transplantation for Type 1 diabetes. *J Diabetes* 2010;2(1):16–22.

33 Chang EN, Scudamore CH, Chung SW. Transplantation: focus on kidney, liver and islet cells. *Can J Surg* 2004;47(2):122–129.

34 Gruessner RW, *et al.* Solitary pancreas transplantation for nonuremic patients with labile insulin-dependent diabetes mellitus. *Transplantation* 1997;64(11):1572–1577.

35 First MR. Immunosuppressive agents and their actions. *Transplant Proc* 2002;34:1369.

36 American Diabetes A. Pancreas transplantation for patients with type 1 diabetes. *Diabetes Care* 2000;23(Suppl 1):S85.

37 Singh RP, *et al.* Do pretransplant C-peptide levels influence outcomes in simultaneous kidney-pancreas transplantation? *Transplant Proc* 2008; 40(2):510–512.

38 Singh RP, *et al.* Outcomes of extended donors in pancreatic transplantation with portal-enteric drainage. *Transplant Proc* 2008;40(2):502–505.

39 Light JA, *et al.* Successful long-term kidney-pancreas transplants regardless of C-peptide status or race. *Transplantation* 2001;71(1):152–154.

40 Sutherland DE, Gruessner AC, Radosevich DM. Transplantation: kidney or kidney-pancreas transplant for the uremic diabetic? *Nat Rev Nephrol* 2009;5(10):554–556.

41 Shrishrimal K, Hart P, Michota F. Managing diabetes in hemodialysis patients: observations and recommendations. *Cleve Clin J Med* 2009;76(11): 649–655.

42 Friedman AL. Appropriateness and timing of kidney and/or pancreas transplants in type 1 and type 2 diabetes. *Adv Ren Replace Ther* 2001;8(1):70–82.

43 Becker BN, *et al.* Simultaneous pancreas-kidney and pancreas transplantation. *Minerva Urol Nefrol* 2002;54(4):213–226.

44 Becker BN, *et al.* Preemptive transplantation for patients with diabetes-related kidney disease. *Arch Intern Med* 2006;166(1):44–48.

45 Reddy KS, *et al.* Long-term survival following simultaneous kidney-pancreas transplantation versus kidney transplantation alone in patients with type 1 diabetes mellitus and renal failure. *Am J Kidney Dis* 2003;41(2):464–470.

46 Reddy KS, *et al.* Long-term survival following simultaneous kidney-pancreas transplantation versus kidney transplantation alone in patients with type 1 diabetes mellitus and renal failure. *Transplant Proc* 2001;33(1–2):1659–1660.

47 Ojo AO, *et al.* The impact of simultaneous pancreas-kidney transplantation on long-term patient survival. *Transplantation* 2001;71(1):82–90.

48 Farney AC, *et al.* Experience in renal and extrarenal transplantation with donation after cardiac death donors with selective use of extracorporeal support. *J Am Coll Surg* 2008;206(5):1028–1037, disc. 1037.

49 Andreoni KA, *et al.* Kidney and pancreas transplantation in the United States, 1996–2005. *Am J Transplant* 2007;7(5 Pt 2):1359–1375.

50 Cohen DJ, *et al.* Kidney and pancreas transplantation in the United States, 1995–2004. *Am J Transplant* 2006;6(5 Pt 2):1153–1169.

51 O'Connor KJ, Delmonico FL. Increasing the supply of kidneys for transplantation. *Semin Dial* 2005;18(6):460–462.

52 Reynoso JF, *et al.* Short- and long-term outcome for living pancreas donors. *J Hepatobiliary Pancreat Sci* 2010;17(2):92–96.

53 Sutherland DE, *et al.* Pancreas transplantation. *Surg Clin North Am* 1986;66(3):557–582.

54 Sutherland DE, Goetz FC, Najarian JS. Intraperitoneal transplantation of immediately vascularized segmental pancreatic grafts without duct ligation. A clinical trial. *Transplantation* 1979;28(6):485–491.

55 Sutherland DE, Goetz FC, Najarian JS. Living-related donor segmental pancreatectomy for transplantation. *Transplant Proc* 1980;12(4 Suppl 2):19–25.

56 Sutherland DE, Baumgartner D, Najarian JS. Free intraperitoneal drainage of segmental pancreas grafts: clinical and experimental observations on technical aspects. *Transplant Proc* 1980;12(4 Suppl 2):26–32.

57 Sutherland DE, *et al.* Lessons learned from more than 1,000 pancreas transplants at a single institution. *Ann Surg* 2001;233(4):463–501.

58 Sutherland DE, Goetz FC, Najarian JS. Clinical segmental pancreas transplantation without duct anastomosis in diabetic renal allograft recipients. *Diabetes* 1980;29(Suppl 1):10–18.

59 American Diabetes Association. Pancreas transplantation for patients with type 1 diabetes. *Diabetes Care* 2000;23(1):117.

60 Nath DS, *et al.* Outcomes of pancreas transplants for patients with type 2 diabetes mellitus. *Clin Transplant* 2005;19(6):792–797.

61 Vandenberg BF, *et al.* Evaluation of diabetic patients for renal and pancreas transplantation: noninvasive screening for coronary artery disease using radionuclide methods. *Transplantation* 1996;62(9):1230–1235.

62 Herzog CA, *et al.* Dobutamine stress echocardiography for the detection of significant coronary artery disease in renal transplant candidates. *Am J Kidney Dis* 1999;33(6):1080–1090.

63 Bates JR, *et al.* Evaluation using dobutamine stress echocardiography in patients with insulin-dependent diabetes mellitus before kidney and/or pancreas transplantation. *Am J Cardiol* 1996;77(2):175–179.

64 Manske CL, *et al*. Coronary revascularisation in insulin-dependent diabetic patients with chronic renal failure. *Lancet* 1992;340(8826):998–1002.

65 Krishnamurthi V, Philosophe B, Bartlett ST. Pancreas transplantation: contemporary surgical techniques. *Urol Clin North Am* 2001;28(4):833–838.

66 Philosophe B, *et al*. Superiority of portal venous drainage over systemic venous drainage in pancreas transplantation: a retrospective study. *Ann Surg* 2001;234(5):689–696.

67 Al-Shurafa HA, *et al*. Innovations in pancreas transplantation. *Saudi Med J* 2002;23(3):265–71.

68 Stratta RJ. Surgical nuances in pancreas transplantation. *Transplant Proc* 2005;37(2):1291–1293.

69 Wee AC, Krishnamurthi V. In: Srinivas TR, Shoskes DA (eds) Pancreas Transplantation: Surgical Techniques; Kidney and Pancreas Transplantation. 2011; New York, NY: Humana Press. pp. 249–258.

70 Stratta RJ, *et al*. Experience with portal-enteric pancreas transplant at the University of Tennessee-Memphis. *Clin Transpl* 1998:239–253.

71 Stratta RJ, *et al*. A prospective comparison of simultaneous kidney-pancreas transplantation with systemic-enteric versus portal-enteric drainage. *Ann Surg* 2001;233(6):740–751.

72 Bartlett ST, *et al*. Pancreas transplantation at the University of Maryland. *Clin Transpl* 1996:271–280.

73 Gruessner AC, Sutherland DE. Pancreas transplant outcomes for United States (US) and non-US cases as reported to the United Network for Organ Sharing (UNOS) and the International Pancreas Transplant Registry (IPTR) as of June 2004. *Clin Transplant* 2005;19(4):433–455.

74 Dubernard JM, *et al*. A new method of preparation of segmental pancreatic grafts for transplantation: trials in dogs and in man. *Surgery* 1978; 84(5):633–639.

75 Traeger J, *et al*. Pancreatic transplantation in man: a new method of pancreas preparation and results on diabetes correction. *Transplant Proc* 1979;11(1):331–335.

76 Kandaswamy R, *et al*. Vascular graft thrombosis after pancreas transplantation: comparison of the FK 506 and cyclosporine eras. *Transplant Proc* 1999;31(1–2):602–603.

77 Benedetti E, *et al*. A prospective randomized clinical trial of perioperative treatment with octreotide in pancreas transplantation. *Am J Surg* 1998;175(1):14–17.

78 Calne RY, *et al*. Cyclosporin A initially as the only immunosuppressant in 34 recipients of cadaveric organs: 32 kidneys, 2 pancreases, and 2 livers. *Lancet* 1979;2(8151):1033–1036.

79 Stratta RJ. Simultaneous use of tacrolimus and mycophenolate mofetil in combined pancreas-kidney transplant recipients: a multi-center report. The FK/MMF Multi-Center Study Group. *Transplant Proc* 1997;29(1–2): 654–655.

80 Gruessner AC, Sutherland DE. Analysis of United States (US) and non-US pancreas transplants as reported to the International Pancreas Transplant Registry (IPTR) and to the United Network for Organ Sharing (UNOS). *Clin Transpl* 1998:53–73.

81 Gruessner RW, *et al*. Mycophenolate mofetil and tacrolimus for induction and maintenance therapy after pancreas transplantation. *Transplant Proc* 1998;30(2):518–520.

82 Singh RP, Stratta RJ. Advances in immunosuppression for pancreas transplantation. *Curr Opin Organ Transplant* 2008;13(1):79–84.

83 Farney A, *et al*. A randomized trial of alemtuzumab vs. anti-thymocyte globulin induction in renal and pancreas transplantation. *Clin Transplant* 2008;22(1):41–49.

84 Thai NL, *et al*. Alemtuzumab induction and tacrolimus monotherapy in pancreas transplantation: one- and two-year outcomes. *Transplantation* 2006;82(12):1621–1624.

85 Starzl TE, *et al*. Tolerogenic immunosuppression for organ transplantation. *Lancet* 2003;361(9368):1502–1510.

86 Schmied BM, *et al*. Immunosuppressive standards in simultaneous kidney-pancreas transplantation. *Clin Transplant* 2006;20(Suppl 17):44–50.

87 Kaufman DB, *et al*. Alemtuzumab induction and prednisone-free maintenance immunotherapy in simultaneous pancreas-kidney transplantation comparison with rabbit antithymocyte globulin induction—long-term results. *Am J Transplant* 2006;6(2):331–339.

88 Aoun M, *et al*. Very early steroid withdrawal in simultaneous pancreas-kidney transplants. *Nephrol Dial Transplant* 2007;22(3):899–905.

89 Fridell JA, *et al*. Steroid withdrawal for pancreas after kidney transplantation in recipients on maintenance prednisone immunosuppression. *Transplantation* 2006;82(3):389–392.

90 Thai NL, *et al*. Pancreas transplantation under alemtuzumab (Campath-1H) and tacrolimus: Correlation between low T-cell responses and infection. *Transplantation* 2006;82(12):1649–1652.

91 Knight RJ, *et al*. Pancreas transplantation utilizing thymoglobulin, sirolimus, and cyclosporine. *Transplantation* 2006;81(8):1101–1105.

92 Gruessner AC, Sutherland DE, Gruessner RW. Pancreas transplantation in the United States: a review. *Curr Opin Organ Transplant* 2010;15(1):93–101.

93 Gruessner AC, Sutherland DE. Report for the international pancreas transplant registry—2000. *Transplant Proc* 2001;33(1–2):1643–1646.

94 Gruessner AC, Sutherland DE. Analysis of United States (US) and non-US pancreas transplants reported to the United network for organ sharing (UNOS) and the international pancreas transplant registry (IPTR) as of October 2001. *Clin Transpl* 2001:41–72.

95 Reddy KS, *et al*. Surgical complications after pancreas transplantation with portal-enteric drainage. *Transplant Proc* 1999;31(1–2):617–618.

96 Gruessner RW, Sutherland DE. Simultaneous kidney and segmental pancreas transplants from living related donors—the first two successful cases. *Transplantation* 1996;61(8):1265–1268.

97 Wuthrich RP. Factor V. Leiden mutation: potential thrombogenic role in renal vein, dialysis graft and transplant vascular thrombosis. *Curr Opin Nephrol Hypertens* 2001;10(3):409–414.

98 Friedman GS, *et al*. Hypercoagulable states in renal transplant candidates: impact of anticoagulation upon incidence of renal allograft thrombosis. *Transplantation* 2001;72(6):1073–1078.

99 Roza AM, Johnson CP, Adams M. Acute torsion of the renal transplant after combined kidney-pancreas transplant. *Transplantation* 1999;67(3):486–488.

100 West MS, *et al*. Renal pedicle torsion after simultaneous kidney-pancreas transplantation. *J Am Coll Surg* 1998;187(1):80–87.

101 Humar A, *et al*. Decreased surgical risks of pancreas transplantation in the modern era. *Ann Surg* 2000;231(2):269–275.

102 Boggi U, *et al*. Total duodenectomy with enteric duct drainage: a rescue operation for duodenal complications occurring after pancreas transplantation. *Am J Transplant* 2010;10(3):692–697.

103 Connolly JE. Pancreatic whole organ transplantation. *Surg Clin North Am* 1978;58(2):383–390.

104 Zibari GB, *et al*. Roux-en-Y venting jejunostomy in pancreatic transplantation: a novel approach to monitor rejection and prevent anastomotic leak. *Clin Transplant* 2000;14(4 Pt 2):380–385.

105 Eckhoff DE, *et al*. Efficacy of 99mTc voiding cystourethrogram for detection of duodenal leaks after pancreas transplantation. *Transplant Proc* 1994; 26(2):462–463.

106 Del Pizzo JJ, *et al*. Urological complications of bladder-drained pancreatic allografts. *Br J Urol* 1998;81(4):543–547.

107 Troppmann C, *et al*. Surgical complications requiring early relaparotomy after pancreas transplantation: a multivariate risk factor and economic impact analysis of the cyclosporine era. *Ann Surg* 1998;227(2):255–268.

108 Kaplan AJ, *et al*. Early operative intervention for urologic complications of kidney-pancreas transplantation. *World J Surg* 1998;22(8):890–894.

109 Kuo PC, *et al*. Solitary pancreas allografts. The role of percutaneous biopsy and standardized histologic grading of rejection. *Arch Surg* 1997;132(1):52–57.

110 Papadimitriou JC, *et al*. Histologic grading scheme for pancreas allograft rejection: application in the differential diagnosis from other pathologic entities. *Transplant Proc* 1998;30(2):267.

111 Klassen DK, *et al*. Pancreas allograft biopsy: safety of percutaneous biopsy-results of a large experience. *Transplantation* 2002;73(4):553–555.

112 Malek SK, *et al*. Percutaneous ultrasound-guided pancreas allograft biopsy: a single-center experience. *Transplant Proc* 2005;37(10):4436–4437.

113 Humar A, *et al*. Technical failures after pancreas transplants: why grafts fail and the risk factors—a multivariate analysis. *Transplantation* 2004; 78(8):1188–1192.

114 Odorico JS, *et al*. Donor factors affecting outcome after pancreas transplantation. *Transplant Proc* 1998;30(2):276–277.

115 Ziaja J, *et al*. Donor-dependent risk factors for early surgical complications after simultaneous pancreas-kidney transplantation. *Transplant Proc* 2011;43(8):3092–3096.

116 Sousa MG, *et al*. Multivariate analysis of risk factors for early loss of pancreas grafts among simultaneous pancreas-kidney transplants. *Transplant Proc* 2010; 42(2):547–551.

117 Lanza RP, Chick WL. Transplantation of encapsulated cells and tissues. *Surgery* 1997;121(1):1–9.

118 Lanza RP, Cooper DK, Chick WL. Xenotransplantation. *Sci Am* 1997;277(1):54–59.

119 Auchincloss H Jr,, Sachs DH. Xenogeneic transplantation. *Annu Rev Immunol* 1998;16:433–470.

120 Shapiro AM, Lakey JR. Future trends in islet cell transplantation. *Diabetes Technol Ther* 2000;2(3):449–452.

121 Furth ME, Atala A. Stem cell sources to treat diabetes. *J Cell Biochem* 2009;106(4):507–511.

122 Orlando G, *et al*. Regenerative medicine as applied to solid organ transplantation: current status and future challenges. *Transpl Int* 2011;24(3):223–232.

6 Allotransplantation of Pancreatic Islets

Maciej T. Juszczak[1] and Paul R.V. Johnson[2,3]

[1] Islet Transplant Programme, Oxford Centre for Diabetes, Endocrinology and Metabolism, and Islet Transplant Research Group, Nuffield Department of Surgical Sciences, University of Oxford, UK
[2] John Radcliffe Hospital, UK
[3] St Edmund Hall, University of Oxford, UK

Introduction

Type-1 diabetes mellitus (T1DM) affects millions of people worldwide and the incidence is rising. The discovery of insulin in 1922 meant that the acute symptoms of T1DM were able to be successfully treated with insulin injections and it is now rarely fatal. However, the chronic, secondary complications of the disease, including neuropathy, retinopathy, and both micro- and macroangiopathy, are now associated with a high personal cost for people with T1DM, including blindness, renal failure, ischemic heart disease, and peripheral vascular disease, as well as an enormous economical cost for Western societies. Novel T1DM therapies therefore aim to stabilize or reverse these secondary complications, or ultimately to prevent these complications altogether by fully reversing T1DM early in the disease. There are a number of potential ways of achieving this, but pancreatic islet transplantation has several key advantages over alternative therapies.

The aim of this chapter is to give an overview of islet allotransplantation, including an outline of: (i) the rationale for this treatment, (ii) the selection and allocation of suitable donor pancreases, (iii) pancreas retrieval and preservation, (iv) human islet isolation, (v) islet culture, (vi) pretransplant graft assessment, (vii) islet recipient selection, (viii) the islet transplant procedure, (ix) post-transplant management, (x) immunosuppression, (xi) the current clinical outcomes, and finally (xii) the ongoing challenges facing the field.

Rationale for islet transplantation

Although the development of the chronic complications of T1DM is multifactorial, there is clear evidence that they are closely linked to the tight glycaemic control. In addition to observations made in studies involving

Abdominal Organ Transplantation: State of the Art, First Edition.
Edited by Nizam Mamode and Raja Kandaswamy.
© 2013 Blackwell Publishing Ltd. Published 2013 by Blackwell Publishing Ltd.

identical twins, studies such as the Diabetes Control and Complications Trial (DCCT) have elegantly demonstrated that intensive insulin regimens resulting in tight glycemic control can significantly reduce the incidence of secondary complications of diabetes compared with conventional insulin treatment [1]. However, the intensive regimens are also associated with life-threatening hypoglycemia [2]. The challenge, therefore, is to develop treatments that are well tolerated, and that ensure restoration of normal glucose homeostasis at an early stage of the disease (i.e. treatments that truly reverse T1DM), in order to prevent the secondary complications from developing, rather than trying to treat these severe conditions once the "horse has already bolted". In addition, as T1DM is principally diagnosed in the first 2 decades of life, any candidate treatment needs to be applicable to children and young adults.

There are a number of potential ways of achieving tight glycemic control. Some of the severe drawbacks of intensive insulin injections can be improved by using insulin pumps, especially if these can be combined with glucose sensors [3,4]. However, this approach still has the disadvantages that it uses exogenous insulin and a mechanical device and that conceptually it is still treating diabetes, rather than truly curing it. The latter can, however, be achieved by the transplantation of insulin-producing tissue, in the form of either a vascularized pancreas transplant or a pancreatic islet cell transplant (ICT). Whole-pancreas transplantation is discussed in detail in Chapter 5, and is a very successful treatment that achieves restoration of normal glucose homeostasis and results in insulin independence rates of up to 85% 1 year post-transplantation. In addition, there is growing evidence that this treatment also reverses the secondary complications of T1DM [5]. However, whole-pancreas transplantation is intrinsically a major surgical procedure, with a high procedure-related morbidity, and mortality rates of up to 4%. The major complications include graft thrombosis, graft pancreatitis, pancreatic fistulae, and pseudocyst formation, which are related to the pancreatic exocrine tissue rather than the β-cell component. Islet transplantation, on the other hand, is a minimally invasive procedure with the same potential to restore normal glucose homeostasis. However, by transplanting only the endocrine component of the pancreas (about 2% of the pancreas mass) as a cellular transplant, this procedure is associated with a very low rate of serious complications. In addition, cellular transplants have the huge potential advantage of being able to be immunomodulated or immunoisolated, thereby preventing the need for long-term immunosuppression (see later). Islet transplantation is potentially widely applicable to children and teenagers. The advantages and disadvantages of whole-pancreas and islet transplantation are compared in Table 6.1.

It is important to emphasize that whole-pancreas transplantation and islet transplantation should be regarded as complementary rather than competitive therapies, and as such, allocation of patients to these two treatments should be tailored to individual patient need. In addition, although the ultimate goal of islet transplantation is to achieve long-term insulin independence, currently the main indication for this treatment in most countries is to treat hypoglycemic unawareness after all conventional

Table 6.1 Characteristics of islet and pancreas transplantation as modalities of β-cell replacement therapy.

	Islet transplant	Pancreas transplant
First performed	1974 (Minneapolis)	1966 (Minneapolis)
Total number of cases	>1,400	>24,000
Donor : recipient ratio	1 : 1–4 : 1	1 : 1
Number of transplants required to achieve therapeutic targets	1–4	1–2
Pretransplant graft testing	Extensive testing possible	No means at present
Preferred mode	IA	SPK
Transplantation procedure	Percutaneous	Laparotomy
Amount of tissue transplanted	0.5–5.0 g	~100 g
Procedure-related complications	Minimal: • bleeding • portal vein thrombosis • biliary tree / gallbladder injury	Significant: • graft thrombosis • graft pancreatitis • anastomotic breakdown • collections • pseudocysts • fistulae • sepsis & peritonitis
Mortality risk	Negligible (~0%)	Moderate (4%)
Insulin independence		
1 year	75%	85%
5 years	15% (<60%)	~70%
Graft function at 5 years	70%	70%

IA, islet alone; SPK, simultaneous pancreas-kidney.

treatments have been exhausted. It is extremely effective at reversing this life-threatening complication of T1DM. However, it must not be forgotten that the potential application of islet transplantation is much greater.

Historical background of islet transplantation

The first attempt to cure diabetes using β-cell replacement was performed in Bristol in 1883, when minced pancreas procured from a sheep was injected into a patient with T1DM [6]. This attempt failed, and with our current knowledge of transplant immunology, this is not surprising! In 1916 the first pancreatic tissue allograft was performed in Newcastle-upon-Tyne by Dr Pybus. In his report, published in *The Lancet* in September 1924, he reported a small reduction in urinary excretion of glucose in one of two diabetic patients whom he transplanted with fragments of pancreatic tissue obtained from human cadaveric donor [7]. Once the association between islets of Langerhans and insulin secretion had been established in the 1920s, scientists started isolating islets from animals in order to study islet physiology, with the hope of treating and curing diabetes. Initially, islet isolation was performed using mechanical disruption, microsurgical dissection, and hand-picking. However, in 1965 Moskalewski developed a new technique of tissue dissociation using a crude preparation of enzymes obtained from culture supernatants from the bacterium *Clostridium histolyticum* and successfully isolated pancreatic islets from a guinea pig [8]. This technique was quickly adopted by Paul Lacy and Mary Kostianovsky in order to isolate islets from rats [9]. It was not until 1974, however, that the first clinical islet allotransplant using isolated islets of Langerhans was performed [10].

Improvements in both islet isolation and islet transplantation occurred over the next few decades, including the development of a semiautomated method for pancreas digestion by Ricordi and the introduction of a large-scale method for islet purification by Lake [11]. However, despite the fact that 494 islet transplants were reported to the International Islet Transplant Registry between 1974 and the end of the 1990s, and the fact that in animal models reversal of diabetes following an islet transplant was almost routine, the results of clinical islet allotransplantation were disappointing, with overall 9% of patients achieving insulin-independence and about 40% achieving partial graft function in the form of C-peptide production (C-peptide levels >0.3 ng/ml) [12].

However, all this changed in 2000 when Shapiro published the results of a small series of islet transplants performed in Edmonton, Canada [13]. Using a steroid-free immunosuppression regime, together with a protocol that involved each patient receiving at least two consecutive islet transplants utilizing large islet numbers, he reported that all seven of his patients had achieved insulin-independence. In addition, the main indication for transplantation in this group was the severe complication of hypoglycemic unawareness, which was also universally reversed by the islet transplants. This landmark publication stimulated the reactivation of other islet-transplant centers across the world, as well as the creation of many new centers. Soon leading groups were reporting insulin-independence rates of 80–85% at 1 year, success rates that were comparable with whole-pancreas transplantation [14].

Donor selection and pancreas allocation

Islet transplantation involves two broad components, namely islet isolation and the islet transplant itself. One of the major challenges of clinical islet transplantation has been to consistently obtain sufficient numbers of high-quality islets to routinely achieve insulin independence after transplantation. There are a number of factors which affect islet-isolation outcome, including donor selection, the variability of pancreas digestion, and the recovery of islet function after isolation and transplantation [15–17].

As with all other forms of allotransplantation, islet transplantation is hindered worldwide by the shortage of organ donors. However, this is compounded by the fact that whole-pancreas teams and islet-transplant teams are principally competing for the same donor organs [18]. Although it is widely stated that the donor criteria for the two modalities are distinctly different, this is based on the criteria of optimal islet yields (islet yields are expressed as both islet numbers and a volume-adjusted islet equivalent (IEq)) rather than the more important measures of pre- and post-transplant islet function. This paradox is exemplified by donor age. Ihm *et al.* have shown nicely that although islet yields increase with donor age, islet function as measured by insulin secretion decreases with age [19]. Therefore, although older donors (>60 years old) are largely excluded from whole-pancreas transplant programs and would be readily available for islet transplants, the reduced islet function and increased apoptosis rates within the islets of these donors mean that they are also largely unsuitable for islet transplantation. There are, however, a few donor factors that favor retrieval for islet transplantation over whole-pancreas transplantation, including high donor body mass index (BMI). These pancreases are often associated with poor vasculature for anastamosing a whole-pancreas graft, but provided the donor has not developed type-2 diabetes, isolated islets from obese donors can have excellent in vitro and in vivo function. The challenge for all forms of transplantation is to be able to expand the donor pool, including finding methods of enabling marginal donors to be used. Table 6.2 summarizes current exclusion criteria for pancreas donors for clinical islet isolation and transplantation in the UK.

Donor age

There are several reports demonstrating that donor age correlates positively with isolation yield and purity [16,17]. Nonetheless, it is now widely accepted that islets isolated from pancreases from donors younger than 55 years demonstrate significantly better function in vitro compared with those of older donors [19]. In addition, the expression of the pancreatic master gene *Pdx1* (whose product, Pdx1, is a pancreatic transcription factor) is decreased with increasing age, while the apoptotic index increases with age. Interestingly, the outcomes of solid-organ transplantation are also better when pancreases from young donors are used. One of the challenges for islet transplantation, however, is that the current methods used for human islet isolation favor the older donor. The pancreases from young donors (<25 years) are very difficult to process, and usually do not yield sufficient numbers of islets for transplantation [15,16]. This seems to be related to the fact that the collagenase enzymes routinely used for pancreas digestion do not efficiently digest the extracellular matrix within the younger pancreas. Encouragingly, newer enzymes seem to be improving isolation outcomes from younger donors.

Body mass index

High body mass is associated with increased deposition of intra-abdominal adipose tissue and the presence of excessive peripancreatic fat. This may result in suboptimal cooling of the pancreas during retrieval and suboptimal preservation. This in turn increases the risk of complications after solid-organ transplantation, including pancreatitis and graft loss. Several studies

Table 6.2 UK exclusion criteria for pancreas donors for clinical islet isolation and transplantation. DBD, donation after brain death; DCD, donation after cardiac death; DSA, donor-specific antibody; ICU, intensive care unit.

Donor criteria

Absolute exclusion criteria

- Donor age <18 or >60 years.
- Diabetes (documented).
- Malignancy, except for primary brain tumors.
- Acute or chronic pancreatitis.
- BMI >40.0.
- Extensive fibrosis or fatty infiltration on inspection at retrieval or at the time of pancreas processing.
- Prolonged cardiac arrest and/or hypotension causing dysfunction of kidney, liver, or pancreas.
- Cold-ischemia time >8 hours (at the time of processing or anticipated arrival to the isolation unit) for DBD and >4 hours for DCD.
- Positive crossmatch or known DSAs.

Relative exclusion criteria

- Damage at retrieval—all pancreases with non-critical damage at retrieval should be inspected in the islet isolation center before being excluded.
- Alcohol abuse—the pancreas should be inspected in the lab to determine morphological features suggestive of chronic alcohol-related pancreatitis, such as extensive fibrosis, calcifications, or fatty infiltrations.
- Suspicion of diabetes or a family history of diabetes—if history is doubtful or unclear, HbA1c levels should be performed and the donor excluded if the level of glycated hemoglobin is greater than 7.0%.
- Nonresolving severe sepsis before donation.
- Prolonged ICU stay (not an independent exclusion factor, although it should be taken into account).
- Prolonged cardiac arrest and significant hypotension requiring vasopressors and inotropes.

have demonstrated that both donor mass and donor BMI correlate with islet isolation outcomes (total islet numbers, as well as IEqs) [15,16,20]. Nevertheless, islets isolated from obese donors have always been treated with some caution as the donors tend to have a type-2 diabetes phenotype. However, recent studies have shown that, provided severe fatty infiltration is not present, fully functional islets can be isolated successfully from donors with a BMI up to 40, and successfully transplanted, even if the donor's glycated hemoglobin is above 7.0% [21].

Cold-ischemia time

Prolonged cold ischemia is detrimental to pancreatic islet isolation. Although it is well documented that cold storage times of up to 8 hours are well tolerated, there is an overall negative correlation between the storage time and islet yield and quality [15,22,23]. Although viable islets can still be isolated from pancreases stored for longer periods of time, the results are inconsistent, and there is a great reluctance to use them for clinical transplantation. A two-layer method (TLM) of pancreas storage has been developed in order to enable pancreases to be effectively stored for long periods (see next section). Although it has some limitations, many groups use this method for suboptimal pancreases with cold ischemia times exceeding 8 hours [24,25].

Pancreas retrieval and preservation

Pancreases for clinical islet isolation should be retrieved in an identical manner to that used for vascularized pancreas transplantation, with the exception of the vessel dissection [26]. The pancreas is therefore removed en bloc with the duodenum and spleen using a no-touch technique. During pancreas dissection, a meticulous technique is required, with avoidance of excessive use of diathermy. Adequate perfusion of the pancreas is of paramount importance and in situ perfusion is often complemented by additional ex vivo perfusion on the back table. During multiorgan retrieval, intravascular cooling is achieved by either aortic or aorto-portal flush. The latter has negative effects on the pancreas and should be avoided. Reduction of the pancreatic core temperature is considered one of the most important steps during pancreas retrieval [27]. Intravascular flush with cold preservation fluid is usually not sufficient and needs to be complemented by external pancreas cooling using copious amounts of ice slush placed in the lesser sac.

Standard preservation techniques involve simple cold storage at 4 °C in University of Wisconsin solution (UW), although some centers use HTK, Celsior, EuroCollins, and Kyoto solutions [28,29]. The pancreas is immersed in at least 300 ml of preservation solution and double-bagged. These conditions allow for preservation of the pancreas for up to 8 hours, with minimal loss of organ quality.

Other preservation protocols have been developed, including the TLM, in which the pancreas is preserved in hypothermia on the interface between oxygen-charged perfluorocarbon and preservation fluid.

Although recent papers have questioned the validity of the TLM, showing very limited tissue penetration of oxygen and of the perfluorocarbon itself [30–32], the 2009 Collaborative Islet Transplant Registry (CITR) report revealed that up to 33% of pancreases retrieved for islet isolation were preserved using this method. Examples of experimental preservation techniques include persufflation of pancreases with gaseous oxygen [33,34] and continuous and pulsatile hypothermic pump perfusion [35]. Thus far, none of these techniques has been used clinically, although recently presented results are encouraging.

Islet isolation procedure

Although groups have been undertaking islet isolation for many years [36–39], the human islet isolation procedure is still far from optimized, providing transplantable yields of islets in less than 50% of pancreas preparations, even in centers with significant experience. The main goal of islet isolation is to extract viable islets that are free from surrounding acinar tissue.

Most centers worldwide use a modified semiautomated technique for human islet isolation described by Ricordi [37]. This involves a two-stage procedure. First, the pancreas digestion stage involves the pancreas being dissociated by a combination of mechanical and enzymatic breakdown, resulting in the islets being liberated from the surrounding exocrine tissue. During this stage, the pancreas is transferred to the isolation facility, where it is dissected and the duodenum, spleen, and superficial fat are removed. The pancreatic duct is identified and cannulated with a venous catheter, and commercially available bacterial collagenase dissolved in Hanks' solution at 4 °C is delivered to the pancreatic parenchyma by intraductal injection, either by a hand-held syringe or by recirculating pumps. The distended pancreas is then divided into a number of pieces and transferred into a metallic or polycarbonate chamber containing marbles or ball bearings. This chamber is connected to a fluid-filled system, in which a medium (usually minimal essential medium, MEM) is circulated at 37 °C. This system allows for accurate control of temperature and fluid flow, which can both be adjusted depending on the progress of digestion. When free islets appear in the digest, the process is stopped by addition of cold buffer into the circuit, and islets are collected into an albumin-enriched medium, commonly containing a cocktail of protease inhibitors.

In the second stage of islet isolation, islet purification, the liberated islets are separated from the exocrine tissue using centrifugation on a density gradient [39–41]. Following incubation of the pancreatic digest for 30–60 minutes in UW, resuspended tissue is loaded on the top of a Ficoll-based continuous gradient within a spinning COBE 2991 cell separator. During centrifugation, tissue fragments and cellular debris accumulate in the top layer (lowest density), big fragments of tissue move towards the bottom of the gradient (highest density), and liberated islets stay in between the two extremes (1.08–1.09 g/l). Purified islets can be transplanted immediately or following a short-term culture.

In order to comply with recent European Union (EU) and US Food and Drug Administration (FDA) regulations, human islet isolation for allotransplantation must now be performed in purpose-built good manufacturing practice (GMP)-grade facilities. As a result, an increasing number of islet transplant networks is developing, in which several centers transplant islets isolated from one core facility. This "hub and spoke" model not only means that the costs can be rationalized, but enables islet-isolation expertise to be centralized and maintained [42].

Islet culture

Although the original Edmonton protocol emphasized the importance of transplanting freshly isolated islets, most groups now recommend a period of 24–48 hours of culture prior to transplantation. Pretransplant culture of clinical preparations has two main purposes. First, it allows for a more thorough assessment of graft quality before the final decision to transplant

[43]. Often an islet preparation can look excellent immediately after islet isolation, but a period of culture can show that in fact cell death was commencing, and after 24 hours of optimal culture the islets may become fragmented and have reduced function. This is particularly the case with large volume islets, in which central necrosis may not be evident immediately [44,45]. It is clearly beneficial to discover this before rather than after the islet transplant. On the other hand, there is clear evidence that a period in culture can also enable islet function to improve, as islets recover from the islet isolation procedure [46]. Second, the logistics of transplanting fresh islets used to mean that patients often had to be admitted in the middle of the night, and the procedure itself became an emergency. A period of islet culture enables the procedure to become semielective and carefully planned.

The specifics of different culture protocols are beyond the scope of this book. However, multiple measures are undertaken in order to limit the damage caused by hypoxic conditions, including low islet seeding density, low depth of medium to facilitate oxygen diffusion, and a wide range of supplements to reduce production and release of pro-inflammatory cytokines and free radicals.

In many centers, gas-permeable bags (similar to the bags used for platelet storage) have been used to facilitate oxygen diffusion to islets in culture. The purification process ends with several fractions containing different degrees of contamination with exocrine tissue. It is a common practice to culture high- and low-purity fractions separately. Purified tissue is placed in large culture flasks ($175\,cm^2$ cultivation area), usually in cell-culture medium, such as CMRL-1066. The seeding density is about $20\,000–30\,000\,IEq$ in $25–30\,ml$ of culture medium. This seeding density, combined with a low depth of culture medium, helps prevent hypoxia in cultured islets. At the end of the culture period, the preparation is reassessed (islet number/loss, viability, microbiological status) and its suitability for transplantation is reevaluated. Although technically possible, prolonged culture is avoided in clinical transplantation and limited to a maximum of 48 hours.

Pretransplant graft assessment

Pretransplant culture of isolated islets allows for assessment of graft quality in terms of morphology, functional status, and sterility. This reduces the chance of poor-quality or contaminated grafts from being transplanted and makes this treatment modality potentially safer than solid organ transplantation. Several parameters are assessed during this process [47–49].

Islet number, size distribution, and islet morphology

Although automated counting is an option, most centers count islets manually [49–51]. This process, while fairly robust, is operator-dependent and the results can differ significantly among centers. In order to identify islets in a suspension, a zinc chelator—dimethylthiocarbazone (Dithizone, DTZ)—is used, which stains islets crimson red [52]. The size distribution of an islet preparation is usually skewed towards small islets; therefore, islet number is not necessarily representative of β-cell volume. In order to adjust for this discrepancy, IEq is used, where 1 IEq represents an islet

150 μm in diameter [53]. The whole population of islets is stratified into size-related groups, with corresponding conversion factors. For instance, for an islet 50–100 μm in diameter, this conversion factor is 0.167, and for an islet 200–250 μm in diameter, it is 3.5. In addition to the number of IEqs, an isolation index (II) is calculated by dividing the number of IEqs by the number of islets. II provides an indication of whether the distribution is skewed towards small or large islets. Analysis of islet morphology determines the degree of fragmentation and cleavage of peri-islet exocrine tissue.

Purity of the preparation

The purity of the preparation is estimated as the percentage of islets compared to acinar tissue. It is subjective, with considerable interassessor variability, but a purity of >50% is required for an islet preparation to be signed off for transplantation in the UK. Indeed, it could be argued that a preparation of <50% is by definition an exocrine transplant!

Islet viability and function

For the purpose of clinical isolation, a fluorescent viability assay is performed [54,55]. This assesses the integrity of the cellular membrane, which in turn is a function of the cell's metabolic state. A principle of this viability test is that dyes such as ethidium bromide or propidium iodide can diffuse into cells and bind to DNA only if cellular-membrane permeability is compromised, as in dead cells. Others, such as fluorescein diacetate or acridine orange, are actively transported inside an intact, living cell and can be either metabolized, resulting in release of fluorescent compound, or bound to DNA. The assessment of islets is performed manually using a fluorescent microscope and is again subject to operator bias.

A glucose-stimulated insulin secretion (GSIS) assay tests the ability of isolated islets to response to glucose stimulation by insulin secretion. Several modifications of this assay exist, but for clinical purposes a static incubation is usually performed, whereby islets are exposed to a baseline (2.5 mM) and/or a stimulatory (25.0 mM) glucose concentration. Following a period of incubation, the insulin concentration before and after stimulation is measured, and the stimulation index (SI) is calculated using the formula:

$$\text{SI} = \text{insulin (stimulated)} \div \text{insulin (basal)}$$

where insulin (stimulated) is the amount of insulin secreted during 1-hour incubation in 25.0 mM glucose medium and insulin (basal) is the amount of insulin secreted during 1-hour incubation in 2.5 mM glucose medium.

An SI in excess of 2 is indicative of a functional preparation. Although this test is used to assess the islet graft, it is usually performed after transplantation. Therefore, its results are not part of the product release criteria listed later.

Microbiological contamination and the presence of endotoxin

Culture of isolated islet allows for a thorough microbiological assessment of the graft prior to transplantation [56,57]. Routine microbiological tests prior to graft release include microscopy and Gram staining, endotoxin levels, and bacterial and fungal cultures. As part of microbiological monitoring, the donor's viral status should be included with product release documentation (cytomegalovirus (CMV) and Epstein–Barr virus (EBV) status in particular) so that the transplanting team can consider appropriate prophylaxis [58,59].

Product release criteria

The current regulations for tissue banks in Europe dictate that clear product release criteria have to be determined and stuck to. In the UK, the following release criteria are used:

- Islet yield >200 000 IEq (although the graft is allocated based on the islet dose in IEq/kg).
- Purity >50% (>30% in the USA).
- Viability >70%.
- Packed cell volume (PCV) <10 ml (recent research from Edmonton suggests that PCV should be limited to 5 ml in order to eliminate the risk of portal-vein thrombosis [60]).
- Microscopy and Gram stain negative.
- Endotoxin level <3-5 EU/ml (values differ between manufacturers and isolation centers).

Islet recipient selection

As islet transplantation develops as a successful treatment, the indications expand and more patients become eligible for its benefits [61]. Overall, however, there are two main groups that are included in the selection criteria worldwide. First and foremost is the small subpopulation of patients suffering from brittle type-1 diabetes, with severe life-threatening hypoglycemic unawareness. These patients benefit enormously from the minimally invasive islet transplants, but are only offered an islet transplant provided that all optimal insulin treatments have been exhausted. The second group is patients with unstable type-1 diabetes in whom a renal graft must be preserved [62]. These transplants can either be performed as a simultaneous islet and kidney transplant (SIK) or as an islet-after-kidney graft (IAK).

It is important to understand that the main goal of islet transplantation is not to achieve insulin-independence but to reverse hypoglycemic unawareness and achieve metabolic stability. Therefore, the expectations of any potential recipient need to be clarified, and all potential recipients should be warned that they may well remain on insulin injections following transplantation. However, although insulin-independence is not the primary goal, it is interesting to note that insulin-independence achieved early after transplantation has been shown to contribute to extended graft longevity and better function [63].

The process of recipient selection requires a multidisciplinary approach and a careful and extensive work-up [64]. Most patients are discussed in the local multidisciplinary team (MDT) meetings, but difficult cases should be discussed in a multicenter MDT meeting to ensure that the decision reached is in the best interests of the patient. The overall aims of the work-up are to ensure that the patient has proven life-threatening hypoglycemic unawareness requiring third-party intervention, to ensure that they are not overtreated with insulin and have received optimal conventional medical treatment, to screen them for premalignant, malignant, or infective conditions that make immunosuppression contraindicated, and to ensure that there is no liver pathology that would prevent a percutaneous, transhepatic intraportal islet infusion.

Confirming life-threatening glycemic instability

All patients with severe hypoglycemia or reduced hypoglycemic awareness over the age of 18 years (no upper age limit) should be considered for islet transplantation if symptoms persist despite optimal medical therapy and no major exclusion criteria are met [65]. The long-term side effects of immunosuppression prevent its application for children and teenagers under 18 years of age at present. It is almost uniformly accepted that patients who experience more than one episode of severe hypoglycemia requiring third-party intervention per year can be considered for ICT, although the incidence of severe hypoglycemic episodes is usually higher. Several scales and scoring systems are used to evaluate hypoglycemia, including the Clark Score, Ryan HYPO Score, and Ryan Lability Index. Evidence of altered hypoglycemia awareness should be demonstrated using a continuous glucose-monitoring system. Individuals with suboptimal glycemic control despite a functional renal graft (IAK) should also be considered for islet transplantation.

Absence of fasting or stimulated C-peptide (with concomitant blood glucose 4 mmol/l) has to be demonstrated before transplantation. It is disputed whether current islet replacement techniques are efficient enough to overcome insulin resistance, which is defined as an insulin requirement of more than 0.7 units/kg body weight/day to achieve an HbA1c <9%. Acceptable maximum insulin requirements vary between transplant centers and programs and can be anything from 0.7 to over 1.0 units/kg body weight. Insulin resistance is proportional to body weight and therefore a potential islet-transplant recipient should weigh less than 80 kg and have a BMI <30 kg/m^2 [66–68].

Screening for contraindications to islet transplantation
Infections and inflammation

Active infection, including hepatitis B or C, HIV, tuberculosis, or aspergillosis within the previous year, constitutes an absolute contraindication to islet transplantation. In several clinical trials, EBV seronegativity is also considered a contraindication to islet transplantation, as it might be associated with a higher risk of acquiring EBV and in turn post-transplant lymphoproliferative disease (PTLD). A positive CMV status of the donor or the recipient is not considered a contraindication to ICT, although it is important to planning CMV prophylaxis following transplantation [58,59,64].

Malignancy

A recent history of malignancy is an absolute contraindication to transplantation; this is true for all except completely resected squamous- or basal-cell carcinoma of the skin and previous malignancies which have been deemed to have been cured (usually >5 years disease-free) [64].

Pregnancy and prospective progeny

Pregnancy or plans for pregnancy (including fatherhood) should be discussed in depth and patients should be warned about potentially harmful effects of immunosuppression. This only constitutes a relative contraindication to ICT.

Immunological considerations

Outside the UK, a panel-reactive antibody (PRA) level greater than 20% (in some centers even 10%) is almost uniformly considered a contraindication to islet transplantation. ICT usually requires two or more transplants to achieve insulin-independence and long-term function; hence the antigen load is significantly higher than after PTA, which in turn increases the risk of further sensitization following graft loss.

Use of steroids

This is a contraindication except in the case of a previous renal graft, or if being used for the treatment of Addison disease where the dose does not exceed 5 mg daily.

Cardiovascular status

Cardiovascular risk is significantly increased in patients with diabetes, and silent coronary-artery disease is relatively common in this population [69]. It is therefore of paramount importance to identify and carefully assess patients at risk. Chest x-ray, electrocardiogram (ECG), and myocardial perfusion scan are performed routinely. Uncorrected myocardial ischemia presenting as unstable angina and recent myocardial infarction (less than 6 months) are absolute contraindications to islet transplantation. Poorly controlled hypertension is also considered a relatively strong contraindication to ICT as it increases risks of cardiovascular and renal complications [64].

Renal function

Due to the fact that the current optimal immunosuppression regimes are nephrotoxic, a careful renal assessment is vital. Prolonged calcineurin-inhibitor and sirolimus-based immunotherapy in patients who already have background diabetic nephropathy may lead to significant deterioration of renal function [70,71], although the risk is small according to recent evidence [63,72,73]. A glomerular filtration rate (GFR) of less than $60 \, ml/minute/1.73 \, m^2$ is a contraindication to islet transplant alone, as is overt proteinuria. An expert nephrologist opinion should be sought in patients with GFR $60-90 \, ml/minute/1.73 \, m^2$. Patients who are IAK candidates will have suboptimal renal function and a degree of macroalbuminuria or even overt proteinuria. For these patients, there are no absolute renal contraindications to islet transplantation, but they should be treated with caution if GFR decreases below 40 ml/minute/1.73 m^2 or serum creatinine is above 175 μmol/l [64].

Liver function

Islet transplantation involves partial, reversible embolization of the distal portal venules. Therefore, hepatic impairment, portal hypertension, and liver hemangioma on baseline ultrasound constitute absolute contraindications to the procedure. A transient deranged hepatic function is commonly observed following islet transplantation (transaminitis) and thus normal liver function prior to the procedure must be confirmed [74]. Persistently elevated liver-function tests above 1.5 times the upper limit of normal are considered a contraindication to islet transplantation [64]. UK guidelines also require the transplant team to consider prophylactic cholecystectomy even for asymptomatic gall-stone disease.

Intestinal absorption

It is very important to take into account any conditions which can cause impairment of intestinal absorption, as immunosuppressive medications (such as tacrolimus) have a narrow therapeutic range, and variation in their blood levels may lead to graft rejection or toxicity. Active gastric or duodenal ulcers, as well as pancreatitis, also preclude listing for islet transplantation.

Hematological considerations

Intraportal islet transplantation is associated with a considerable risk of post-procedural bleed and portal-vein thrombosis. Thus coagulopathies, low platelet count ($<$150 000), anticoagulant, and antiplatelet therapy (with the exception of aspirin) should be considered contraindications to islet transplantation using a percutaneous, transhepatic approach. Several agents used in transplantation, including mycophenolate, cotrimoxazole, and alemtuzumab, are known to cause severe leucopoenia with neutropoenia and even pancytopoenia. Neutropoenic sepsis in not seen as often as in patients with malignancies, but precautions should nevertheless be taken to avoid unnecessary risk. Preexisting benign conditions causing leucopoenia, neutropoenia, or pancytopoenia should be treated with caution, but are not an absolute contraindication to islet transplantation.

Choosing between solid-organ and cell therapy

It has already been emphasized that whole-pancreas transplantation alone and islet transplantation alone represent different approaches to β-cell replacement therapy and should be treated as complementary rather than competitive. Both treatment modalities have their advantages and disadvantages and should be considered on a case-to-case basis. Nevertheless, there are situations where pancreas transplant is more appropriate. These include, for instance, patients eligible for simultaneous pancreas–kidney (SPK) transplantation, aged less than 50, and without major perioperative risks precluding whole-organ transplantation. Patient choice should also be taken into account.

Islet transplantation procedure

Once the suitability of the islet graft for transplantation has been confirmed, islets are allocated to the most suitable recipient. The islets are matched for blood group, and although allocation schemes differ between countries, most schemes take into account time on the waiting list, previous islet transplants, immunological status, and the brittleness of the diabetes.

There are no absolute predictors of the outcome of islet transplantation, although a number of factors have been identified as correlating with insulin independence [17,67,75–78]. Two widely accepted criteria are the total number of islets transplanted and the pretransplant insulin requirement. As a general rule of thumb, a minimum dose of 5000 IEq/kg should be used for a first transplant, whereas the second should be no less than 4000 IEq/kg. This rule should be observed very strictly, as transplantation of a suboptimal islet graft with subsequent graft failure has major immunological implications for the patient in terms of sensitization. Conversely, it is extremely difficult to apply this rule very stringently when dealing with a sensitized patient, in whom the chance of getting another transplantable preparation is rather low. In such cases, it is worth considering transplantation even of a less pure, lower-than-recommended dose if the patient can benefit from this intervention. Alternatively, a vascularized pancreas transplant should be considered.

Patients undergoing an islet transplant are placed on a tight insulin sliding scale and given broad-spectrum antibiotics. They are also given their induction immunosuppression. Other medication is given according to the local protocol.

Islet infusion

Islet allotransplants are normally infused via the portal vein. In most centers, this is done using the percutaneous transhepatic radiological approach, although a minilaparotomy with cannulation of one of the minor tributaries of the portal vein is considered an option in patients with very difficult radiological access [63,79,80]. In very difficult cases, it is also worth considering a transjugular approach.

The transhepatic procedure is performed under local anesthesia, with sedation by interventional radiologist. The patient is starved prior to this procedure, in case a general anesthesia is required, and therefore an insulin sliding scale is started on admission. Access to the portal vein is gained percutaneously under ultrasound and fluoroscopic control. The portal vein is cannulated retrograde with a 5–7 French catheter. Islet transplantation is performed by gravitational infusion using a bag technique [81]. This is considered safer than the previously used hand-controlled injection, although infusion times are now considerably longer.

Infusion of islets can trigger the coagulation cascade and cause portal-vein thrombosis. It has been shown that the risk of portal-vein thrombosis increases with increased PCV and high opening portal pressure [60]. Therefore, prior to infusion, islet suspension is supplemented with unfractionated heparin. It is also essential to monitor portal-venous pressure throughout the procedure to ensure it remains within a safe range. A baseline portal pressure is established prior to islet infusion. An opening pressure of up to 13 mm Hg can be considered safe for this procedure, whereas portal pressures between 13 and 17 mm Hg should be treated with caution. Portal pressure above 17 mm Hg should be considered an absolute contraindication to intraportal islet transplantation. If the PCV exceeds 5 ml, portal pressure is monitored every 2–3 minutes. Increase of portal pressure to above twice the opening pressure or above an absolute value of 17 mm Hg is an indication to put the infusion on hold for a few minutes. If the vital parameters do not change and the portal pressure decreases spontaneously, the infusion can be restarted. If, on the other hand, portal pressure stays high or rises, the possibility of portal-vein thrombosis should be considered and appropriate management instigated.

Following infusion, a closing portal pressure is measured and recorded and the catheter is removed from the portal vein.

Initial series of islet transplants resulted in a significant number of procedure-related bleeds. Use of heparin, low platelet counts, and lack of hemostatic devices in the cannulation tract were identified as risk factors. As a result, plugging devices were introduced, and it is now a standard clinical practice to plug the tract formed by insertion of the catheter with hemostatic gels and coils [82].

Post-transplant management

The success of islet transplantation depends on three major factors: the infusion of an optimal islet graft, the selection of a suitable islet recipient, and careful and well-organized post-transplant care. It is extremely important that a multidisciplinary team involving both islet-transplant specialists, transplant surgeons, and diabetologists is involved in the care of these patients. The constant support from other specialists, including nephrologists, is also vital.

Immediate post-transplant management
On return from the radiology department, patients require 24 hours' bed rest, with the initial 4 hours lying down on the right side to reduce the chance of bleeding from the puncture site. Vital signs are monitored frequently for the first 6 hours. Patients continue to be nil-by-mouth for the first 4 hours after the procedure and are on clear fluids thereafter for the first 24 hours after the procedure in order to facilitate maintenance of stable glycemia in the early post-transplant period.

Tight glucose control following islet transplantation is thought to be beneficial for β-cell survival and islet engraftment [68]. An insulin sliding scale should be used in the post-transplant period for 24–48 hours after islet infusion in order to maintain body mass between 4 and 7 mmol/l. After the initial 24 hours, insulin requirements are assessed and patients are restarted on their pretransplant regimen with an adjusted insulin dose.

Intraportal islet infusion may trigger portal-vein thrombosis and therefore appropriate prophylaxis should be used in the peritransplant period (unfractionated heparin 5000 units twice daily subcutaneously, or low-molecular-weight heparin of choice). Some centers use therapeutic anti-coagulation (a continuous infusion of unfractionated heparin with target activated partial thromboplastin time (APTT) of 70–90 seconds) instead of subcutaneous heparin [68]. The infusion is usually discontinued after 48 hours and patients are switched to low-molecular-weight heparin, which continues for 7 days. The impact of islet transplantation on coagulation and the effectiveness of prophylaxis should be assessed by thromboelastogram performed within the first 24 hours after islet infusion.

Although the incidence of portal-vein thrombosis peaks 24 hours after transplantation, it can occur for up to 35 days after infusion. It is important to detect and treat these complications early, and an ultrasound scan is routinely performed 24 hours after transplantation. Further imaging depends on the clinical picture and indications.

The minimally invasive nature of the procedure allows for a quick and uneventful recovery. Patients only stay in the hospital for 2–3 days, during which time both the insulin requirement and the immunosuppressive regime are established.

Outpatient follow-up

The initial outpatient follow-up is necessarily intensive. Recipients should be seen by transplant and diabetes teams to ensure both aspects of patient care are covered sufficiently. In the early post-transplant period, like solid-organ-transplant recipients, patients are seen at very regular, short intervals. This is beneficial for the patients as optimization of immunosuppressive therapy and assessment of early graft function are performed at this stage. With time, the frequency and intensity of the follow-up decreases. A typical follow-up schedule is presented in this section:

Follow-up clinic visits after discharge

Twice a week for 4 weeks, fortnightly for a further 3 months, then monthly for up to 1 year (or when indicated), and every 3 months thereafter.

Diabetic monitoring and assessment of graft function

Home finger-prick tests taken seven times a day for the first month, then four times a day until 3 months post-transplant. Intensified body-mass monitoring is continued beyond 3 months only if clinically indicated (this includes continuous glucose-monitoring systems (CGMS)).

Metabolic assessment

A mixed-meal tolerance test (MMTT) is performed at 1, 3, 6, and 12 months after transplantation. C-peptide and HbA1c levels, ICA and anti-GAD antibodies, and retinal screening are all performed at the same time as MMTT.

Immunological assessment

Monitoring of the formation of donor-specific antibodies is carried out. Blood samples for tissue-typing are taken at 48 hours, 7 days, 14 days, 4 weeks, and then at every clinic appointment.

Immunosuppression

Although it is anticipated that cell transplantation will be amenable to immunoalteration or immunoisolation strategies in the future, contrary to common belief, islets are not in themselves immunoprivileged, and certainly are no less susceptible to allogeneic response and rejection than other organs. Therefore, recipients require the same level of immunosuppression as after solid-organ transplantation. Moreover, the management of post-transplant immunosuppression is complicated by the fact that it is extremely difficult to monitor islet rejection.

Following a publication by Shapiro and colleagues in 1998, which showed that the combination of calcineurin inhibitors (CNI) and steroids has a direct β-cell toxicity [83], significant changes were introduced to islet immunosuppressive protocols, rendering regimes steroid-free and CNI-sparing [13,84]. Indeed, the so-called Edmonton protocol transformed the outcomes of clinical islet transplantation.

The edmonton protocol

This original immunosuppressive protocol made it possible to achieve long-term function following islet transplantation. It includes daclizumab as an induction agent and dual maintenance therapy consisting of tacrolimus (trough levels 4–6 ng/ml) and rapamycin (trough levels 12–15 ng/ml in the first 3 months, followed by 10–12 ng/ml thereafter). Initial results showed 80% insulin-independence after 1 year, but long-term results were disappointing, with insulin-independence rates below 20% after 3 years. Interestingly, the Lille group reported 60% 3-year insulin-independence in patients on the same immunosuppressive regimen. It is thought that this effect might be attributed to rapid achievement of insulin-independence due to early supplemental islet infusions, rather than immunosuppression or a total islet dose.

It is not surprising therefore that the Edmonton protocol was the most common immunosuppressive regimen (51.2% of all transplant recipients) until 2008, as reported by the CITR [85]. Subsequently this changed, with an increasing use of lymphocyte-depleting agents and mycophenylate mofetil (MMF), and the proportion of patients on alternative immunosuppressive regimens increased to over 88%. Tacrolimus-based protocols, especially in combination with MMF, seem to be on the rise (70 and 31% of protocols, respectively), whereas Sirolimus seems to be losing its role (67% of protocols) compared with trends reported by the CITR in 2006 (74% of all protocols; 83 verus 98% of all patients). Similarly, daclizumab (41% of all immunosuppression protocols), used for induction in the original Edmonton protocol, is now being replaced by antithymocyte globulin (ATG) and Campath (43 and 7% of all immunosuppression protocols, respectively). Indeed, the results of islet transplants in which Campath has been used as the induction agent are very encouraging [86].

Further changes to immunosuppressive regimens are expected in the near future, with novel biological agents being introduced and evaluated in clinical trials, and cell-based therapies, aiming to induce tolerance, being developed.

Summary of clinical outcomes

The outcomes of clinical islet transplantation should be analyzed in the context of the main therapeutic goals of the procedure, namely resolution of life-threatening hypoglycemic unawareness and stabilization of glycemic control as measured by HbA1c. Composite metabolic outcomes are also useful. Thus several metabolic assays and scoring systems have been validated for the assessment of islet grafts. The most widely used include the intravenous glucose tolerance test (IVGTT), arginine-stimulation test (AST), MMTT, SUITO index, and, perhaps most commonly, the beta score [63,87–90]. The other important outcome measure is the achievement of primary graft function [63]; this is defined as achieving a beta score ≥ 7 [88] (the beta score is a clinical scoring system describing the function of the islet graft; it takes into account glycemic control, treatment of diabetes, and insulin secretion; scores range from 0 (graft failure) to 8 (excellent function)). In contrast, primary graft nonfunction is defined as undetectable fasting or stimulated C-peptide levels at any time point between 7 and 31 days (inclusive) after islet transplantation. Transplant clinicians often insist on appraisal of islet transplantation using the same outcomes as solid-organ transplantation, which includes the incidence of insulin-independence. Indeed, clinical experiments and small clinical trials studying the efficacy of islet transplantation now report insulin-independence as their primary outcome.

Results reported by the CITR show that in 2009 the overall incidence of sustained graft function was 77% after the first 6 months, 66% after 1 year, and 45% at 3 years [85]. These results are significantly better than those achieved before the year 2000, when the 3-year incidence of sustained graft function was reported by the Islet Transplant Registry (Giessen) to be only 19% [12]. The CITR reported the overall incidence of insulin-independence, irrespective of the number of infusions, to be 55% at month 6 post-last infusion, declining steadily to reach only 16% in year 4. It is noteworthy that there is a significant disparity between the outcomes from experienced centers and those from less experienced ones. Noticeably, a recent report by the Lille group indicated a higher incidence of both sustained graft function and insulin-independence if good primary function was achieved. Their overall 3-year incidence of insulin-independence was 57%, but reached 78% for patients who achieved good primary graft function [63]. Both the Minneapolis and the Edmonton groups have also reported a higher incidence of sustained graft function and insulin-independence in patients receiving insulin–heparin infusion in the immediate post-transplant period [67,68,91].

Restoration of insulin production, even in the absence of insulin-independence, has been shown to improve overall glycemic control and thus prevent episodes of hypoglycemia and restore hypoglycemic awareness. The incidence of life-threatening hypoglycemia decreases dramatically following islet transplantation [92]. The proportion of patients free from severe hypoglycemic episodes increases from about 2% pretransplant to over 65% at 1 year, then steadily decreases over the follow-up to less than 25% at 4 years. These data are based on well-documented cases; it has to be emphasized that ~50% of data for 4-year follow-up were missing from the CITR 2009 analysis.

It is too early to make definitive comments about the influence of islet transplantation on the chronic complications of diabetes. However, some small studies have attempted to assess the effect of islet transplantation on cardiovascular [93] and renal function [72,94,95], and the effect of normalization of glucose metabolism on the progression of retinopathy [95–98]. Although very promising, these results should be interpreted with caution due to the small number of subjects and the uncontrolled nature of the studies.

Ongoing challenges in islet transplantation

While the field of islet transplantation has made enormous strides over the past decade, there are still a number of key challenges preventing it from becoming widely available, and from achieving its ultimate goal of treating children. Major challenges include: the shortage and poor quality of pancreas donors [18,99]; the inconsistency of islet isolation; loss of islets during culture, islet transportation, and following transplantation [46,100–102]; determination of the ideal anatomical site for islet implantation [103,104]; difficulties with imaging [105–107]; immunological monitoring of islet grafts [108,109]; and, importantly, prevention of the need for immunosuppression (in order to make the procedure applicable to young children [110]).

Ongoing research in these areas has led to a number of improvements in transplant protocols. Most notably, in recent years islet isolation has benefited from the introduction of new, improved digestion enzymes and enzyme mixtures [111–115]. Further research in this field is required, concentrating specifically on a composition of the extracellular matrix at the exocrine/endocrine interface. Better understanding of the islet's microenvironment would help inform the design of novel strategies to enable more efficient liberation of islets, resulting in the efficient utilization of every available pancreas.

Although great progress has been made since 2000, transplant centers still report a significant islet loss during even short periods of pretransplant culture. Hypoxia seems to be the main factor causing a substantial graft loss [44], and a lot of effort has been dedicated to its prevention by the introduction of oxygen-permeable bags [116,117] and supplemental oxygen, and by attempts to use biologically inert oxygen-carrying agents such as perfluorocarbons [118,119]. Research in this area continues, in order to ensure optimal conditions for the storage and transportation of isolated islets [102].

Over recent years, much research has been conducted into graft loss after intraportal islet transplantation. Since Gray and Korsgren independently described the in vitro phenomenon now termed the "instant blood-mediated inflammatory reaction" (IBMIR) [120–123], several studies have suggested that this reaction may have a major impact on the survival of intraportally transplanted islets [124]. Unfortunately, not all studies have been conclusive. A recent publication by the Edmonton group analyzing IBMIR as an independent factor affecting successful engraftment did not provide definitive answers [68]. The post-transplant graft loss is also a consequence of a failure to engraft. It has been proposed that the liver may be an unfavorable transplant site for islets, and may not promote graft revascularization and remodeling. Alternative transplantation sites (such as muscle, bone-marrow cavity, spleen, omental pouch, and kidney subcapsular space) have been investigated for a potential clinical application, with some promising results [103,104].

With the introduction of new biological induction agents, immunosuppressive regimens have evolved to produce excellent long-term outcomes. Nevertheless, most protocols still include diabetogeneic compounds (CNIs) that are suspected to cause graft loss in the long term. Progression to CNI-free protocols would therefore be desirable [84,125,126], and new potential biological agents, such as belatacept, should be able to open this avenue [127–129].

Another approach is to avoid immunosuppression by creating a state of tolerance in the recipient and to create either a mechanical (micro- and macrocapsules) or a biological (endothelial cell-coating) barrier between isolated islets and the recipient's immune system [102,130–134].

A shortage of good-quality donor pancreases is one of the major obstacles hampering islet transplantation. In an effort to obtain a sustainable source of insulin-producing cells, several alternative sources have been proposed. These include xenogeneic islets (e.g. genetically modified porcine islets), stem cells, pluripotent mesenchymal cells, and bone marrow. The search for an elusive β-cell progenitor cell still continues [135,136]. Although considerable success has been achieved in this area, the main factors delaying the clinical application of xenografts are the great difficulty of crossing xenogeneic immunological barriers and the fear of transmissible diseases [137,138]. On the other hand, stem-cell research and tissue engineering should allow for the creation of a bioartificial pancreas in the near future. Unfortunately, the genetic instability of engineered graft material has repeatedly resulted in a high incidence of malignant transformation. Before islet stem-cells can be used clinically, this major obstacle needs to be overcome.

References

1 DCCT Research Group. The effect of intensive treatment of diabetes on the development and progression of long-term complications in insulin-dependent diabetes mellitus. *N Engl J Med* 1993;329(14):977–986.

2 DCCT Research Group. Hypoglycemia in the Diabetes Control and Complications Trial. *Diabetes* 1997;46(2):271–286.

3 Vaddiraju S, Burgess DJ, Tomazos I, Jain FC, Papadimitrakopoulos F. Technologies for continuous glucose monitoring: current problems and future promises. *J Diabetes Sci Technol* 2010;4(6):1540–1562.

4 Hovorka, Roman. Closed-loop insulin delivery: from bench to clinical practice. *Nat Rev Endocrinol* 2011;7(7):385–395.

5 Jahansouz C, Kumer SC, Ellenbogen M, Brayman KL. Evolution of beta cell replacement therapy in diabetes mellitus: pancreas transplantation. *Diabetes Technol Ther* 2011;13:395–418.

6 Williams W. Notes on diabetes treated with extract and by grafts of sheep's pancreas. *BMJ* 1984;2(1771):1303–1304.

7 Pybus FC. Notes on suprarenal and pancreatic grafting. *Lancet* 1924;ii: 550–551.

8 Moskalewski , Stanislaw. Isolation and culture of the islets of Langerhans of the guinea pig. *Gen Comp Endocrinol* 1965;44(Jun):342–353.

9 Lacy PE, Kostianovsky M. Method for the isolation of intact islets of Langerhans from the rat pancreas. *Diabetes* 1967;16(1):35–39.

10 Najarian JS, Sutherland DE, Matas AJ, Steffes MW, Simmons RL, Goetz FC. Human islet transplantation: a preliminary report. *Transplant Proc* 1977;9(1): 233–236.

11 Lake SP, Bassett PD, Larkins A, Revell J, Walczak K, Chamberlain J, Rumford GM, London NJ, Veitch PS, Bell PR. Large-scale purification of human islets utilizing discontinuous albumin gradient on IBM 2991 cell separator. *Diabetes* 1989;38(Suppl 1(Jan)):143–145.

12 Brendel MD, Hering BJ, *Schultz AO*, Bretzel RG. Newsletter of the International Islet Transplant Registry. 2001.

13 Shapiro AM, Lakey JR, Ryan EA, Korbutt GS, Toth E, Warnock GL, Kneteman NM, Rajotte RV. Islet transplantation in seven patients with type 1 diabetes mellitus using a glucocorticoid-free immunosuppressive regimen. *N Engl J Med* 2000;343(4):230–238.

14 Shapiro AMJ, Ricordi C, Hering B. Edmonton's islet success has indeed been replicated elsewhere. *Lancet* 2003;362(9391):1242.

15 Ponte GM, Pileggi A, Messinger S, Alejandro A, Ichii H, Baidal DA, Khan A, Ricordi C, Goss JA, Alejandro R. Toward maximizing the success rates of human islet isolation: influence of donor and isolation factors. *Cell Transplant* 2007; 16(6):595–607.

16 Hanley SC, Paraskevas S, Rosenberg L. Donor and isolation variables predicting human islet isolation success. *Transplantation* 2008:85(7):950–955.

17 Niclauss N, Bosco D, Morel P, Demuylder-Mischler S, Brault C, Milliat-Guittard L, Colin C, Parnaud G, Muller YD, Giovannoni L, Meier R, Toso C,

Badet L, Benhamou P-Y, Berney T. Influence of donor age on islet isolation and transplantation outcome. *Transplantation* 2011:91(3);360–366.

18 Berney T, Johnson PRV. Donor pancreata: evolving approaches to organ allocation for whole pancreas versus islet transplantation. *Transplantation* 2010;90(3):238–243.

19 Ihm S-H, Matsumoto I, Sawada T, Nakano M, Zhang HJ, Ansite JD, Sutherland DER, Hering B-HJ. Effect of donor age on function of isolated human islets. *Diabetes* 2006;55(5):1361–1368.

20 Brandhorst H, Brandhorst D, Hering BJ, Federlin K, Bretzel RG. Body mass index of pancreatic donors: a decisive factor for human islet isolation. *Exp Clin Endocrinol Diabetes* 1995;103(Suppl 2):23–26.

21 Koh A, Kin T, Imes S, Shapiro AMJ, Senior P. Islets isolated from donors with elevated HbA1c can be successfully transplanted. *Transplantation* 2008;86(11):1622–1624.

22 Benhamou PY, Watt PC, Mullen Y, Ingles S, Watanabe Y, Nomura Y, Hober C, Miyamoto M, Kenmochi T, Passaro EP. Human islet isolation in 104 consecutive cases. Factors affecting isolation success. *Transplantation* 1994;57(12):1804–1810.

23 Lakey LR, Warnock GL, Rajotte RV, Suarez-Alamazor ME, Ao Z, Shapiro AM, Kneteman NM. Variables in organ donors that affect the recovery of human islets of Langerhans. *Transplantation* 1996;61(7):1047–1053.

24 Tsujimura T, Kuroda Y, Kin T, Avila JG, Rajotte RV, Korbutt GS, Ryan EA, Shapiro AMJ, Lakey JRT. Human islet transplantation from pancreases with prolonged cold ischemia using additional preservation by the two-layer (UW solution/perfluorochemical) cold-storage method. *Transplantation* 2002;74(12):1687–1691.

25 Kuehtreiber WM, Ho LT, Kamireddy A, Yacoub JAW, Scharp DW. Islet isolation from human pancreas with extended cold ischemia time. *Transplant Proc* 2010;42(6):2027–2031.

26 Ridgway D, Manas D, Shaw J, White S. Preservation of the donor pancreas for whole pancreas and islet transplantation. *Clin Transplant* 2010;24(1):1–19.

27 Lakey JRT, Kneteman NM, Rajotte RV, Wu DC, Bigam D, Shapiro AMJ. Effect of core pancreas temperature during cadaveric procurement on human islet isolation and functional viability. *Transplantation* 2002;73(7):1106–1110.

28 Baertschiger RM, Berney T, Morel P. Organ preservation in pancreas and islet transplantation. *Curr Opin Organ Transplant* 2008;13(1):59–66.

29 Caballero-Corbalan J, Brandhorst H, Malm H, Felldin M, Foss A, Salmela K, Tibell A, Tufveson G, Korsgren O, Brandhorst D. Using HTK for Prolonged Pancreas Preservation Prior to Human Islet Isolation. *J Surg Res* 2011;Mar.

30 Papas KK, Hering BJ, Guenther L, Gunther L, Rappel MJ, Colton CK, Avgoustiniatos ES. Pancreas oxygenation is limited during preservation with the two-layer method. *Transplant Proc* 2005;37(8):3501–3504.

31 Caballero-Corbalan J, Eich T, Lundgren T, Foss A, Felldin M, Kallen R, Salmela K, Tibell A, Tufveson G, Korsgren O, Brandhorst D. No beneficial effect of two-layer storage compared with UW-storage on human islet isolation and transplantation. *Transplantation* 2007;84(7):864–869.

32 Agrawal A, Bainbridge A, Powis S, Fuller B, Cady EB, Davidson BR. 31-phosphorus magnetic resonance spectroscopy for dynamic assessment of adenosine triphosphate levels in pancreas preserved by the two-layer method. *Transplant Proc* 2011;43(5):1801–1809.

33 Scott WE 3rd, Weegman BP, Ferrer-Fabrega J, Stein SA, Anazawa T, Kirchner VA, Rizzari MD, Stone J, Matsumoto S, Hammer BE, Balamurugan AN, Kidder LS, Suszynski TM, Avgoustiniatos ES, Stone SG, Tempelman LA, Sutherland DER, Hering BJ, Papas KK. Pancreas oxygen persufflation increases ATP levels as shown by nuclear magnetic resonance. *Transplant Proc* 2010;42(6):2011–2015.

34 Scott WE 3rd, O'Brien TD, Ferrer-Fabrega J, Avgoustiniatos ES, Weegman BP, Anazawa T, Matsumoto S, Kirchner VA, Rizzari MD, Murtaugh MP, Suszynski TM, Aasheim T, Kidder LS, Hammer BE, Stone SG, Tempelman LA, Sutherland DER, Hering BJ, Papas KK. Persufflation improves pancreas preservation when compared with the two-layer method. *Transplant Proc* 2010;42(6):2016–2019.

35 Karcz M, Cook HT, Sibbons P, Gray C, Dorling A, Papalois V. An ex-vivo model for hypothermic pulsatile perfusion of porcine pancreata: hemodynamic and morphologic characteristics. *Exp Clin Transplant* 2010;8(1):55–60.

36 Gray DW, McShane P, Grant A, Morris PJ. A method for isolation of islets of Langerhans from the human pancreas. *Diabetes* 1984;33(11):1055–1061.

37 Ricordi C, Lacy PE, Finke EH, Olack BJ, Scharp DW. Automated method for isolation of human pancreatic islets. *Diabetes* 1988;37(4):413–420.

38 Kenmochi T, Miyamoto M, Une S, Nakagawa Y, Moldovan S, Navarro RA, Benhamou PY, Brunicardi FC, Mullen Y. Improved quality and yield of islets isolated from human pancreata using a two-step digestion method. *Pancreas* 2000;20(2):184–190.

39 Friberg AS Stahle M, Brandhorst H, Korsgren O, Brandhorst D. Human islet separation utilizing a closed automated purification system. *Cell Transplant* 2008;17(12):1305–1313.

40 Anazawa T, Matsumoto S, Yonekawa Y, Loganathan G, Wilhelm JJ, Soltani SM, Papas KK, Sutherland DER, Hering BJ, Balamurugan AN. Prediction of pancreatic tissue densities by an analytical test gradient system before purification maximizes human islet recovery for islet autotransplantation/allotransplantation. *Transplantation* 2011;91(5):508–514.

41 Mita A, Ricordi C, Miki A, Barker S, Khan A, Alvarez A, Hashikura Y, Miyagawa S, Ichii H. Purification method using iodixanol (OptiPrep)-based density gradient significantly reduces cytokine chemokine production from human islet preparations, leading to prolonged beta-cell survival during pretransplantation culture. *Transplant Proc* 2009;41(1):314–315.

42 Kempf M-C, Andres A, Morel P, Benhamou P-Y, Bayle F, Kessler L, Badet L, Thivolet C, Penfornis A, Renoult E, Brun J-M, Atlan C, Renard E, Colin C, Milliat-Guittard L, Pernin N, Demuylder-Mischler S, Toso C, Bosco D, Berney T; GRAGIL Group. Logistics and transplant coordination activity in the GRAGIL Swiss-French multicenter network of islet transplantation. *Transplantation* 2005;79(9):1200–1205.

43 Berney T. Islet culture and counter-culture. Transpl Int 2008;Nov.

44 Giuliani M, Moritz W, Bodmer E, Dindo D, Kugelmeier P, Lehmann R, Gassmann M, Groscurth P, Weber M. Central necrosis in isolated hypoxic human pancreatic islets: evidence for postisolation ischemia. *Cell Transplant* 2005;14(1):67–76.

45 Lehmann R, Zuellig RA, Kugelmeier P, Baenninger PB, Moritz W, Perren A, Clavien P-A, Weber M, Spinas GA. Superiority of small islets in human islet transplantation. *Diabetes* 2007;56(3):594–603.

46 Kerr-Conte J, Vandewalle B, Moerman E, Lukowiak B, Gmyr V, Arnalsteen L, Caiazzo R, Sterkers A, Hubert T, Vantyghem MC, Pattou F. Upgrading

pretransplant human islet culture technology requires human serum combined with media renewal. *Transplantation* 2010;89(9):1154–1160.

47 Shapiro AMJ, Ricordi C, Hering BJ, Auchincloss H, Lindblad R, Robertson RP, Secchi A, Brendel MD, Berney T, Brennan DC, Cagliero E, Alejandro R, Ryan EA, DiMercurio B, Morel P, Polonsky KS, Reems J-A, Bretzel RG, Bertuzzi F, Froud T, Kandaswamy R, Sutherland DER, Eisenbarth G, Segal M, Preiksaitis J, Korbutt GS, Barton FB, Viviano L, Seyfert-Margolis V, Bluestone J, Lakey JRT. International trial of the Edmonton protocol for islet transplantation. *N Engl J Med* 2006;355(13):1318–1330.

48 Hanson MS, Park EE, Sears ML, Greenwood KK, Danobeitia JS, Hullett DA, Fernandez LA. A simplified approach to human islet quality assessment. *Transplantation* 2010;89(10):1178–1188.

49 Kissler HJ, Niland JC, Olack B, Ricordi C, Hering BJ, Naji A, Kandeel F, Oberholzer J, Fernandez L, Contreras J, Stiller T, Sowinski J, Kaufman DB. Validation of methodologies for quantifying isolated human islets: an Islet Cell Resources study. *Clin Transplant* 2010;24(2):236–242.

50 Niclauss N, Sgroi A, Morel P, Baertschiger R, Armanet M, Wojtusciszyn A, Parnaud G, Muller Y, Berney T, Bosco D. Computer-assisted digital image analysis to quantify the mass and purity of isolated human islets before transplantation. *Transplantation* 2008;86(11):1603–1609.

51 Friberg AS, Brandhorst H, Buchwald P, Goto M, Ricordi C, Brandhorst D, Korsgren O. Quantification of the islet product: presentation of a standard-ized current good manufacturing practices compliant system with minimal variability. *Transplantation* 2011;91(6):677–683.

52 Latif ZA, Noel J, Alejandro R. A simple method of staining fresh and cultured islets. *Transplantation* 1988;45(4):827–830.

53 Bretzel RG, Alejandro R, Hering BJ, van Suylichem PT, Ricordi C. Clinical islet transplantation: guidelines for islet quality control. *Transplant Proc* 1994; 26(2):388–392.

54 Miyamoto M, Morimoto Y, Nozawa Y, Balamurugan AN, Xu B, Inoue K. Establishment of fluorescein diacetate and ethidium bromide (FDAEB) assay for quality assessment of isolated islets. *Cell Transplant* 2000;9(5):681–686.

55 Gray DW, Morris PJ. The use of fluorescein diacetate and ethidium bromide as a viability stain for isolated islets of Langerhans. *Stain Technol* 1987;62(6):373–381.

56 Bucher P, Oberholzer J, Bosco D, Mathe Z, Toso C, Buhler LH, Berney T, Morel P. Microbial surveillance during human pancreatic islet isolation. *Transpl Int* 2005;18(5):584–589.

57 Kin T, Rosichuk S, Shapiro AMJ, Lakey JRT. Detection of microbial contam-ination during human islet isolation. *Cell Transplant* 2007;16(1):9–13.

58 Cure P, Pileggi A, Faradji RN, Baidal DA, Froud T, Selvaggi G, Ricordi C, Alejandro R. Cytomegalovirus infection in a recipient of solitary allogeneic islets. *Am J Transplant* 2006;6(5 Pt 1):1089–1090.

59 Gala-Lopez BL, Senior PA, Koh A, Kashkoush SM, Kawahara T, Kin T, Humar A, Shapiro AMJ. Late cytomegalovirus transmission and impact of T-depletion in clinical islet transplantation. *Am J Transplant* 2011;Sep.

60 Kawahara T, Kin T, Kashkoush S, G-Lopez B, Bigam DL, Kneteman NM, Koh A, Senior PA, Shapiro AMJ. Portal vein thrombosis is a potentially preventable complication in clinical islet transplantation. *Am J Transplant* 2011.;Aug.

61 Robertson RP, Davis C, Larsen J, Stratta R, Sutherland DER; American Diabetes Association. Pancreas and islet transplantation in type 1 diabetes. *Diabetes Care* 2006;29(4):935.

62 Cure P, Pileggi A, Froud T, Messinger S, Faradji RN, Baidal DA, Cardani R, Curry A, Poggioli R, Pugliese A, Betancourt A, Esquenazi V, Ciancio G, Selvaggi G, Burke GW 3rd, Ricordi C, Alejandro R. Improved metabolic control and quality of life in seven patients with type 1 diabetes following islet after kidney transplantation. *Transplantation* 2008;85(6):801–812.

63 Vantyghem M-C, Kerr-Conte J, Arnalsteen L, Sergent G, Defrance F, Gmyr V, Declerck N, Raverdy V, Vandewalle B, Pigny P, Noel C, Pattou F. Primary graft function, metabolic control, and graft survival after islet transplantation. *Diabetes Care* 2009;32(8):1473–1478.

64 UK Islet Transplant Consortium. UK Islet Allotransplant Selection, Assessment and Follow-up Criteria. 2010.

65 Ryan EA, Shandro T, Green K, Paty BW, Senior PA, Bigam D, Shapiro AMJ, Vantyghem M-C. Assessment of the severity of hypoglycemia and glycemic lability in type 1 diabetic subjects undergoing islet transplantation. *Diabetes* 2004;53(4):955–962.

66 Shapiro AMJ, Ricordi C. Unraveling the secrets of single donor success in islet transplantation. *Am J Transplant* 2004;4(3):295–298.

67 Hering BJ, Kandaswamy R, Ansite JD, Eckman PM, Nakano M, Sawada T, Matsumoto I, Ihm S-H, Zhang H-J, Parkey J, Hunter DW, Sutherland DER. Single-donor, marginal-dose islet transplantation in patients with type 1 diabetes. *JAMA* 2005;293(7):830–835.

68 Koh A, Senior P, Salam A, Kin T, Imes S, Dinyari P, Malcolm A, Toso C, Nilsson B, Korsgren O, Shapiro AMJ. Insulin-heparin infusions peritransplant substantially improve single-donor clinical islet transplant success. *Transplantation* 2010;89(4):465–471.

69 Senior PA, Welsh RC, McDonald CG, Paty BW, Shapiro AMJ, Ryan EA. Coronary artery disease is common in nonuremic, asymptomatic type 1 diabetic islet transplant candidates. *Diabetes Care* 2005;28(4):866–872.

70 Ryan EA, Lakey JR, Rajotte RV, Korbutt GS, Kin T, Imes S, Rabinovitch A, Elliott JF, Bigam D, Kneteman NM, Warnock GL, Larsen I, Shapiro AM. Clinical outcomes and insulin secretion after islet transplantation with the Edmonton protocol. *Diabetes* 2001;50(4):710–719.

71 Senior PA, Paty BW, Cockfield SM, Ryan EA, Shapiro AMJ. Proteinuria developing after clinical islet transplantation resolves with sirolimus withdrawal and increased tacrolimus dosing. *Am J Transplant* 2005;5(9):2318–2323.

72 Fung MA, Warnock GL, Ao Z, Keown P, Meloche M, Shapiro RJ, Ho S, Worsley D, Meneilly GS, Al Ghofaili K, Kozak SE, Tong SO, Trinh M, Blackburn L, Kozak RM, Fensom BA, Thompson DM. The effect of medical therapy and islet cell transplantation on diabetic nephropathy: an interim report. *Transplantation* 2007;84(1):17–22.

73 Leitao CB, Cure P, Messinger S, Pileggi A, Lenz O, Froud T, Faradji RN, Selvaggi G, Kupin, Warren R, Camillo AR. Stable renal function after islet transplantation: importance of patient selection and aggressive clinical management. *Transplantation* 2009;87(5):681–688.

74 Barshes NR, Lee TC, Goodpastor SE, Balkrishnan R, Schock AP, Mote A, Brunicardi FC, Alejandro R, Ricordi C, Goss JA. Transaminitis after pancreatic islet transplantation. *J Am Coll Surg* 2005;200(3):353–361.

75 Hering BJ. Achieving and maintaining insulin independence in human islet transplant recipients. *Transplantation* 2005;79(10):1296–1297.

76 Nano R, Clissi B, Melzi R, Calori G, Maffi P, Antonioli B, Marzorati S, Aldrighetti L, Freschi M, Grochowiecki T, Socci C, Secchi A, Carlo VD,

Bonifacio E, Bertuzzi F. Islet isolation for allotransplantation: variables associated with successful islet yield and graft function. *Diabetologia* 2005;48(5):906–912.

77 Goto M, Holgersson J, Kumagai-Braesch M, Korsgren O. The ADP/ATP ratio: a novel predictive assay for quality assessment of isolated pancreatic islets. *Am J Transplant* 2006;6(10):2483–2487.

78 Bertuzzi F, Ricordi C. Prediction of clinical outcome in islet allotransplantation. *Diabetes Care* 2007;30(2):410–417.

79 Casey JJ, Lakey JR, Ryan EA, Paty BW, Owen R, O'Kelly K, Nanji S, Rajotte RV, Korbutt GS, Bigam D, Kneteman NN, Shapiro AM. Portal venous pressure changes after sequential clinical islet transplantation. *Transplantation* 2002;74(7):913–915.

80 Goss JA, Soltes G, Goodpastor SE, Barth M, Lam R, Brunicardi FC, Froud T, Alejandro R, Ricordi C. Pancreatic islet transplantation: the radiographic approach. *Transplantation* 2003;76(1):199–203.

81 Baidal DA, Froud T, Ferreira JV, Khan A, Alejandro R, Ricordi C. The bag method for islet cell infusion. *Cell Transplant* 2003;12(7):809–813.

82 Villiger P, Ryan EA, Owen R, O'Kelly K, Oberholzer J, Al Saif F, Kin T, Wang H, Larsen I, Blitz SL, Menon V, Senior P, Bigam DL, Paty B, Kneteman NM, Lakey JRT, Shapiro AMJ. Prevention of bleeding after islet transplantation: lessons learned from a multivariate analysis of 132 cases at a single institution. *Am J Transplant* 2005;5(12):2992–2998.

83 Shapiro AM, Hao E, Lakey JR, Finegood D, Rajotte RV, Kneteman NM. Diabetogenic synergism in canine islet autografts from cyclosporine and steroids in combination. *Transplant Proc* 1998;30(2):527.

84 Shapiro AMJ. State of the art of clinical islet transplantation and novel protocols of immunosuppression. *Curr Diab Rep* 2011;11(5):345–354.

85 Appel M, Hering B. CITR (Collaborative Islet Transplant Registry) Sixth Annual Report. 2009.

86 Froud T, Baidal DA, Faradji R, Cure P, Mineo D, Selvaggi G, Kenyon NS, Ricordi C, Alejandro R. Islet transplantation with alemtuzumab induction and calcineurin-free maintenance immunosuppression results in improved short-and long-term outcomes. *Transplantation* 2008;86(12):1695– 1701.

87 Street CN, Lakey JRT, Shapiro AMJ, Imes S, Rajotte RV, Ryan EA, Lyon JG, Kin T, Avila J, Tsujimura T, Korbutt GS. Islet graft assessment in the Edmonton Protocol: implications for predicting long-term clinical outcome. *Diabetes* 2004;53(12):3107–3114.

88 Ryan EA, Paty BW, Senior PA, Lakey JRT, Bigam D, Shapiro AMJ. Beta-score: an assessment of beta-cell function after islet transplantation. *Diabetes Care* 2005;28(2):343–347.

89 Baidal DA, Faradji RN, Messinger S, Froud T, Monroy K, Ricordi C, Alejandro R. Early metabolic markers of islet allograft dysfunction. *Transplantation* 2009;87(5):689–697.

90 Matsumoto S, Noguchi H, Hatanaka N, Shimoda M, Kobayashi N, Jackson A, Onaca N, Naziruddin B, Levy MF. SUITO index for evaluation of efficacy of single donor islet transplantation. *Cell Transplant* 2009;18(5):557–562.

91 Bellin MD, Kandaswamy R, Parkey J, Zhang H-J, Liu B, Ihm SH, Ansite JD, Witson J, Bansal-Pakala P, Balamurugan AN, Papas KK, Papas K, Sutherland DER, Moran A, Hering BJ. Prolonged insulin independence after islet allotransplants in recipients with type 1 diabetes. *Am J Transplant* 2008;8(11):2463–2470.

92 Leitao CB, Tharavanij T, Cure P, Pileggi A, Baidal DA, Ricordi C, Alejandro R. Restoration of hypoglycemia awareness after islet transplantation. *Diabetes Care* 2008;31(11):2113–2115.

93 Fiorina P, Folli F, Bertuzzi F, Maffi P, Finzi G, Venturini M, Socci C, Davalli A, Orsenigo E, Monti L, Falqui L, Uccella S, Rosa SL, Usellini L, Properzi G, Carlo VD, Maschio AD, Capella C, Secchi A. Long-term beneficial effect of islet transplantation on diabetic macro-/microangiopathy in type 1 diabetic kidney-transplanted patients. *Diabetes Care* 2003;26(4):1129–1136.

94 Fiorina P, Folli F, Zerbini G, Maffi P, Gremizzi C, Carlo VD, Socci C, Bertuzzi F, Kashgarian M, Secchi A. Islet transplantation is associated with improvement of renal function among uremic patients with type I diabetes mellitus and kidney transplants. *J Am Soc Nephrol* 2003;14(8):2150–2158.

95 Thompson DM, Meloche M, Ao Z, Paty B, Keown P, Shapiro RJ, Ho S, Worsley D, Fung M, Meneilly G, Begg I, Al Mehthel M, Kondi J, Harris C, Fensom B, Kozak SE, Tong SO, Trinh M, Warnock GL. Reduced progression of diabetic microvascular complications with islet cell transplantation compared with intensive medical therapy. *Transplantation* 2011;91(3):373–378.

96 Lee TC, Barshes NR, O'Mahony CA, Nguyen L, Brunicardi FC, Ricordi C, Alejandro R, Schock AP, Mote A, Goss JA. The effect of pancreatic islet transplantation on progression of diabetic retinopathy and neuropathy. *Transplant Proc* 2005;37(5):2263–2265.

97 Lee TC, Barshes NR, Agee EE, O'Mahoney CA, Brunicardi FC, Goss JA. The effect of whole organ pancreas transplantation and PIT on diabetic complications. *Curr Diab Rep* 2006;6(4):323–327.

98 Thompson DM, Begg IS, Harris C, Ao Z, Fung MA, Meloche RM, Keown P, Meneilly GS, Shapiro RJ, Ho S, Dawson KG, Al Ghofaili K, Al Riyami L, Al Mehthel M, Kozak SE, Tong SO, Warnock GL. Reduced progression of diabetic retinopathy after islet cell transplantation compared with intensive medical therapy. *Transplantation* 2008;85(10):1400–1405.

99 Shapiro AMJ, Sutherland DER. The new deceased donor pancreas allocation schema: do the recommendations go far enough? *Transplantation* 2007;83(9):1151–1152.

100 Murdoch TB, McGhee-Wilson D, Shapiro AMJ, Lakey JRT. Methods of human islet culture for transplantation. *Cell Transplant* 2004;13(6):605–617.

101 Kin T, Senior P, O'Gorman D, Richer B, Salam A, Shapiro AMJ. Risk factors for islet loss during culture prior to transplantation. *Transpl Int* 2008;21(11):1029–1035.

102 Daoud J, Rosenberg L, Tabrizian M. Pancreatic islet culture and preservation strategies: advances, challenges, and future outlook. *Cell Transplant* 2010;19(12):1523–1535.

103 van der Windt DJ, Echeverri GJ, Ijzermans JNM, Cooper DKC. The choice of anatomical site for islet transplantation. *Cell Transplant* 2008;17(9): 1005–1014.

104 Rajab A. Islet transplantation: alternative sites. *Curr Diab Rep* 2010;10(5): 332–337.

105 Low G, Hussein N, Owen RJT, Toso C, Patel VH, Bhargava R, Shapiro AMJ. Role of imaging in clinical islet transplantation. *Radiographics* 2010; 30(2):353–366.

106 Saudek F, Jirak D, Girman P, Herynek V, Dezortova M, Kriz J, Peregrin J, Berkova Z, Zacharovova K, Hajek M. Magnetic resonance imaging of pancreatic islets transplanted into the liver in humans. *Transplantation* 2010; 90(12):1602–1606.

107 Eriksson O, Alavi A. Imaging the islet graft by positron emission tomography. *Eur J Nucl Med Mol Imaging* 2011;Sep.

108 Toso C, Pawlick R, Lacotte S, Edgar R, Davis J, McCall M, Morel P, Mentha G, Berney T, Shapiro AMJ. Detecting rejection after mouse islet transplantation utilizing islet protein-stimulated ELISPOT. *Cell Transplant* 2011; 20(6):955–962.

109 Lacotte S, Berney T, Shapiro AMJ, Toso C. Immune monitoring of pancreatic islet graft: towards a better understanding, detection and treatment of harmful events. *Expert Opin Biol Ther* 2011;11(1):55–66.

110 Verrotti A, Chiuri RM, Blasetti A, Mohn A, Chiarelli F. Treatment options for paediatric diabetes. *Expert Opin Pharmacother* 2010;11(15):2483–2495.

111 O'Gorman D, Kin T, Imes S, Pawlick R, Senior P, Shapiro AMJ. Comparison of human islet isolation outcomes using a new mammalian tissue-free enzyme versus collagenase NB-1. *Transplantation* 2010;90(3):255–259.

112 Caballero-Corbalan J, Friberg AS, Brandhorst H, Nilsson B, Andersson HH, Felldin M, Foss A, Salmela K, Tibell A, Tufveson G, Korsgren O, Brandhorst D. Vitacyte collagenase HA: a novel enzyme blend for efficient human islet isolation. *Transplantation* 2009;88(12):1400–1402.

113 Caballero-Corbalan J, Brandhorst H, Asif S, Korsgren O, Engelse M, de Koning E, Pattou F, Kerr-Conte J, Brandhorst D. Mammalian tissue-free liberase: a new GMP-graded enzyme blend for human islet isolation. *Transplantation* 2010;90(3):332–333.

114 Brandhorst H, Friberg A, Nilsson B, Andersson HH, Felldin M, Foss A, Salmela K, Tibell A, Tufveson G, Korsgren O, Brandhorst D. Large-scale comparison of Liberase HI and collagenase NB1 utilized for human islet isolation. *Cell Transplant* 2010;19(1):3–8.

115 McCarthy RC, Breite AG, Green ML, Dwulet FE. Tissue dissociation enzymes for isolating human islets for transplantation: factors to consider in setting enzyme acceptance criteria. *Transplantation* 2011;91(2):137–145.

116 Papas KK, Avgoustiniatos ES, Tempelman LA, Weir GC, Colton CK, Pisania A, Rappel MJ, Friberg AS, Bauer AC, Hering BJ. High-density culture of human islets on top of silicone rubber membranes. *Transplant Proc* 2005;37(8):3412–3414.

117 Avgoustiniatos ES, Hering BJ, Rozak PR, Wilson JR, Tempelman LA, Balamurugan AN, Welch DP, Weegman BP, Suszynski TM, Papas KK. Commercially available gas-permeable cell culture bags may not prevent anoxia in cultured or shipped islets. *Transplant Proc* 2008;40(2):395–400.

118 Juszczak MT, Elsadig A, Kumar A, Muzyamba M, Pawelec K, Powis SH, Press M. Use of perfluorodecalin for pancreatic islet culture prior to transplantation: a liquid-liquid interface culture system—preliminary report. *Cell Transplant* 2011;20(2):323–332.

119 Maillard E, Juszczak MT, Clark A, Hughes SJ, Gray DRW, Johnson PRV. Perfluorodecalin-enriched fibrin matrix for human islet culture. *Biomaterials* 2011;Sep.

120 Bennet W, Sundberg B, Groth CG, Brendel MD, Brandhorst D, Brandhorst H, Bretzel RG, Elgue G, Larsson R, Nilsson B, Korsgren O. Incompatibility between human blood and isolated islets of Langerhans: a finding with implications for clinical intraportal islet transplantation? *Diabetes* 1999;48(10):1907–1914.

121 Bennet W, Groth CG, Larsson R, Nilsson B, Korsgren O. Isolated human islets trigger an instant blood mediated inflammatory reaction: implications for intraportal islet transplantation as a treatment for patients with type 1 diabetes. *Ups J Med Sci* 2000;105(2):125–133.

122 Badet L, Titus T, Metzen E, Handa A, McShane P, Chang L-W, Giangrande P, Gray DWR. The interaction between primate blood and mouse islets induces accelerated clotting with islet destruction. *Xenotransplantation* 2002;9(2):91–96.

123 Titus TT, Horton PJ, Badet L, Handa A, Chang L, Agarwal A, McShane P, Giangrande P, Gray DWR. Adverse outcome of human islet-allogeneic blood interaction. *Transplantation* 2003;75(8):1317–1322.

124 Nilsson B, Ekdahl KN, Korsgren O. Control of instant blood-mediated inflammatory reaction to improve islets of Langerhans engraftment. *Curr Opin Organ Transplant* 2011;Oct.

125 Posselt AM, Bellin MD, Tavakol M, Szot GL, Frassetto LA, Masharani U, Kerlan RK, Fong L, Vincenti FG, Hering BJ, Bluestone JA, Stock PG. Islet transplantation in type 1 diabetics using an immunosuppressive protocol based on the anti-LFA-1 antibody efalizumab. *Am J Transplant* 2010;10(8): 1870–1880.

126 Posselt AM, Szot GL, Frassetto LA, Masharani U, Stock PG. Clinical islet transplantation at the University of California, San Francisco. *Clin Transpl* 2010;2010:235–243.

127 Truong W, Plester JC, Hancock WW, Merani S, Murphy TL, Murphy KM, Kaye J, Anderson CC, Shapiro AMJ. Combined coinhibitory and costimulatory modulation with anti-BTLA and CTLA4Ig facilitates tolerance in murine islet allografts. *Am J Transplant* 2007;7(12):2663–2674.

128 Truong W, Plester JC, Hancock WW, Kaye J, Merani S, Murphy KM, Murphy TL, Anderson CC, Shapiro AMJ. Negative and positive co-signaling with anti-BTLA (PJ196) and CTLA4Ig prolongs islet allograft survival. *Transplantation* 2007;84(10):1368–1372.

129 Emamaullee JA, Davis J, Pawlick R, Toso C, Merani S, Cai S-X, Tseng B, Shapiro AMJ. Caspase inhibitor therapy synergizes with costimulation blockade to promote indefinite islet allograft survival. *Diabetes* 2010;59(6):1469–1477.

130 Boninsegna S, Bosetti P, Carturan G, Dellagiacoma G, Dal Monte R, Rossi M. Encapsulation of individual pancreatic islets by sol-gel SiO2: a novel procedure for perspective cellular grafts. *J Biotechnol* 2003;100(3):277–286.

131 Calafiore R, Basta G, Luca G, Calvitti M, Calabrese G, Racanicchi L, Macchiarulo G, Mancuso F, Guido L, Brunetti P. Grafts of microencapsulated pancreatic islet cells for the therapy of diabetes mellitus in non-immunosuppressed animals. *Biotechnol Appl Biochem* 2004;39(Pt 2):159–164.

132 Johansson U, Elgue G, Nilsson B, Korsgren O. Composite islet-endothelial cell grafts: a novel approach to counteract innate immunity in islet transplantation. *Am J Transplant* 2005;5(11):2632–2639.

133 Kim H-I, Yu JE, Lee SY, Sul AY, Jang MS, Rashid MA, Park SG, Kim SJ, Park C-G, Kim JH, Park KS. The effect of composite pig islet-human endothelial cell grafts on the instant blood-mediated inflammatory reaction. *Cell Transplant* 2009;18(1):31–37.

134 Borg DJ, Bonifacio E. The use of biomaterials in islet transplantation. *Curr Diab Rep* 2011;11(5):434–444.

135 Hanley S, Rosenberg L. Islet-derived progenitors as a source of in vitro islet regeneration. *Methods Mol Biol* 2009;482:371–385.

136 Godfrey KJ, Mathew B, Bulman JC, Shah O, Clement S, Gallicano GI. Stem cell-based treatments for Type 1 diabetes mellitus: bone marrow, embryonic,

hepatic, pancreatic and induced pluripotent stem cells. *Diabet Med* 2011;Aug.

137 Abrahante JE, Martins K, Papas KK, Hering BJ, Schuurman H-J, Murtaugh MP. Microbiological safety of porcine islets: comparison with source pig. *Xenotransplantation* 2011;18(2):88–93.

138 Elliott RB; Living Cell Technologies. Towards xenotransplantation of pig islets in the clinic. *Curr Opin Organ Transplant* 2011;16(2):195–200.

7 Novel Cell Therapies in Transplantation

Paul G. Shiels[1], Karen S. Stevenson[2], Marc Gingell Littlejohn[2], and Marc Clancy[3]

[1] Department of Surgery, University of Glasgow, Western Infirmary Glasgow, UK
[2] Institute of Cancer Sciences, College of Medical, Veterinary and Life Sciences, University of Glasgow, UK
[3] University of Glasgow, School of Medicine, UK

Introduction

Human organs have a limited capacity for repairing themselves. This capacity declines as a function of increasing chronological age, driven by a cocktail of biological, psychological, and sociological stressors that can accelerate organ degeneration. Both transplant-recipient survival and donor organ function are affected by these processes. Novel therapies to tackle this are manifold, but typically limited in effect.

Solid-organ transplants replace diseased organs with biologically newer, healthier whole organs, but this strategy is inherently limited. The requirement for an individual with healthy organs to die or to undergo major surgery in order for an organ to be replaced is the central limiting paradox of whole-organ transplantation. Stem-cell treatments represent perhaps the most exciting and most logical of the many ways in which this clinical problem is being addressed. The isolation and propagation of stem-cell lines promised a more permanent and potent method of repair or regeneration of damaged tissue or organs. Indeed, at the time of James Thompson's description of the first embryonic stem-cell lines in 1998 [1], solid-organ transplantation had been established for nearly 3 decades, and the step to having perfect, quality-controlled neo-organs on a shelf ready for surgical implantation appeared small. Initial perceptions have seemingly underestimated the quantum leap from single multipotent stem cell to functioning organ.

The holy grail of cell-based tissue-engineering approaches remains the growth of functional (and ideally tolerant) neo-organs that can spontaneously, or surgically, assimilate into the body and fulfill the role of a diseased organ. While pluripotent cell lines of infinite proliferative capacity have reliably been made to form cardiac myocytes, hepatocytes, and many of the different renal-specific cell types, few have been directed into a neo-organ of adequate function to establish a role in clinical practice, and none in the fields currently managed by major abdominal-organ transplants.

Abdominal Organ Transplantation: State of the Art, First Edition.
Edited by Nizam Mamode and Raja Kandaswamy.
© 2013 Blackwell Publishing Ltd. Published 2013 by Blackwell Publishing Ltd.

Therapeutic applications of novel cell lines are far more advanced in immunomodulation and the augmentation of tissue repair. These protection/repair therapies have already shown clinical benefit and have direct implications for the treatment of age-related disease. Since these approaches are well advanced in clinical trials and therefore likely to find a clinical role in the current abdominal-transplant field, this chapter focuses principally on the potential of cell sources to protect or repair diseased organs. The use of stem cells to grow functional, clinically useful tissue for the treatment of the diseases currently best managed by abdominal-organ transplants remains entirely experimental. Progress and barriers to clinical use are thus also discussed.

Defined stem-cell populations for clinical application

Despite this great promise, the use of regenerative medicine to effect repair of solid organs and tissues is still in its infancy. The type(s) of cell, or cell population, required to effect functional recovery remains to be defined, as do the mechanism, delivery system, and indeed cell numbers to achieve this.

A range of cell types have been touted and tried as candidates for therapeutic use. These include embryo stem cells (ESCs), hematopoietic stem cells (HSCs), multipotent stromal cells (MSCs), endothelial progenitor cells (EPCs), and organ-specific resident stem/progenitor cells, which are known to contribute to solid-organ tissue repair. The individual merits of these cells have been reviewed elsewhere [2]. Currently, their use is limited, but the field is developing rapidly and early clinical trials for solid-organ repair are ongoing.

The main focus is on adult cell sources, since the use of ESCs remains dogged by social and scientific uncertainty, due to moral/ethical issues and basic technical hurdles. The latter include control of the directed differentiation of ESCs and the prevention of neoplasia or tissue dysfunction post-transplant. Most current clinical potential resides with the use of adult cell types, such as MSCs. To date, only MSCs have been applied successfully in both experimental solid-organ transplantation and clinical studies. These are discussed next, with reference to clinical applications in transplantation.

Multipotent stromal cells

MSCs were initially described over 30 years ago by Friedenstein *et al.* as a bone-marrow-derived mononuclear cell population which exhibited a fibroblast-like morphology when cultured ex vivo on an adherent substrate, such as plastic [3]. MSCs are present in a wide range of adult tissues and exhibit the capacity to be differentiated into multiple specialized cell types from all three germ layers. They also demonstrate immunomodulatory properties, though how this is achieved remains undefined (for a detailed review, see [4]). As such, they are of interest due to their capacity to make cells suitable for transplantation. Their isolation is straightforward, either in tissue culture or by fluorescence-activated cell sorting (FACS), where they can be identified by cytotype.

Recent clinical trials have tested the capacity of MSCs to treat cardiac, renal, and liver damage, as noted later in this chapter. What remains unclear, however, is the mode of action of such cells. It is uncertain whether these cells contribute to tissue building via direct differentiation into tissue-specific cells, modulate immune-mediated damage at the site of injury, or even provide trophic support for tissue regeneration [5]. Even the characterization of these cells is contentious.

A basic set of criteria for MSCs has been proposed by the International Society for Cellular Therapy (ISCT) [6]. This appears to function well in practice:

1. Adherence in vivo when grown on plastic.
2. Expression of a specific cell-surface marker phenotype comprising ($CD73^+$ $CD90^+$ $CD105^+$ $CD34^-$ $CD45^-$ $CD11b^-$ $CD14^-$ $CD19^-$ $CD79a^-$ $HLA-DR^-$).
3. Differentiation potential to osteogenic, chondrogenic, and adipogenic lineages.

One key question at this juncture is whether the phenotype and properties exhibited by MSCs in vitro are maintained in vivo. MSCs in vitro typically grow as an adherent monolayer, with a distinct immuno phenotype. When grown under nonadherent conditions, this phenotype changes and the cells grow in spherical clusters. This has been proposed to promote intercellular interactions, although that remains to be demonstrated formally [7].

Some findings, however, suggest that MSCs offer exciting therapeutic potential for organ transplantation. Secretory factors derived from MSCs have been demonstrated to have both pro-angiogenic and anti-inflammatory effects, which might be used to assist in solid-organ and cellular transplantation. Furthermore, MSCs grown in the presence of pro-inflammatory cytokines also display enhanced immunosuppressive effects, which might be exploited to aid transplant success [8–10]. The immunomodulatory effect of MSCs appears to be dose-dependent and independent of the major histocompatibility complex (MHC) and mediation by antigen-presenting cells or regulatory T cells [11,12].

MSCs and solid-organ transplantation

Following on the heels of a range of rodent studies demonstrating that transplanted MSCs can improve tissue damage [13], clinical trials are underway. Currently, only three phase-III clinical trials have been concluded. These comprise trials for graft-versus-host disease (GVHD), Crohns disease, and perianal fistula. As such they are not yet directly relevant to abdominal-organ transplantation, and the therapeutic approach is immunomodulatory, rather than building/repairing tissue architecture (i.e. directly replacing damaged tissue in a failing organ).

Early-stage trials for use with solid organs are limited. Initial findings from a safety-and-clinical-feasibility study [14] comprising autologous MSC administration in two subjects receiving living related-donor kidneys showed that 1 year post-transplant the patients had stable graft function and, significantly, an enlargement of the regulatory T-cell (Treg) pool in the peripheral blood, with a concomitant inhibition of memory T cells. This has demonstrated the feasibility of translating beneficial immunomodulatory findings from rodent models into a human clinical setting, though caution, based on the low power of the study, is still advised.

Ongoing trials using MSC to aid outcome in liver–renal transplantation continue at a number of centers, with results awaited. Promising results on deriving liver and biliary cells in vitro using rodent progenitor cells have already been reported [15], though these have yet to translate into clinical practice, as deriving human equivalents has proven problematic.

Recently, a significant technical breakthrough was reported with the identification of adult nephron progenitors capable of kidney regeneration in zebrafish [16]. The authors provided a proof of principal that transplantation of single aggregates comprising 10–30 progenitor cells is sufficient to engraft adults and generate multiple nephrons. The identification of these cells opens up an avenue to isolating or engineering the equivalent cells in humans and developing novel renal regenerative therapies.

Acute hepatic failure and inborn errors of metabolism affecting the liver can also be treated successfully with hepatocyte transplantation alone [17–19]. This technique is feasible for bridging to orthotopic liver transplantation or for long-term correction of underlying metabolic deficiencies. Hepatocytes can be used fresh or cryopreserved, making them readily available for short-notice administration. The main disadvantage of this technique is the limited source of cells which are isolated from unused donor tissue. In addition, these unused organs are of inferior quality, and this is reflected in the function of the isolated hepatocytes. Intraportal injection is the preferred method of delivery, but alternative routes such as splenic intraparenchymal injection and the peritoneal cavity have been considered [20]. Fetal hepatocytes and hepatic stem-cell transplantation are currently experimental but may prove to be an invaluable therapeutic alternative.

How MSCs might work

How MSCs work in clinical trials and animal models is still debated. Any paracrine effect mediated by the secretion of growth factors remains problematic, as the speed of efficacy, duration of immunomodulation, and extent of tissue repair cannot readily be accounted for. This, principally, is due to the transient existence of MSCs following in vivo administration and different syngeneic and allogeneic effects in transplantation models [21,22].

Recent data from Stevenson et al. shed light some light on this, as even in a xenotransplant setting paracrine effects can invoke developmental recapitulation during organ regeneration [23]. This is discussed more fully later, with reference to pathfinder cells.

Considerations for solid-organ transplantation

Given the convincing in vivo demonstrations of the immunosuppresive effects of MSCs, phase-I clinical trials for the treatment of a range of diseases are already underway. However, their use in organ transplantation still has many potential pitfalls.

First, allogeneic MSCs may induce memory responses, leading to accelerated graft rejection, which would not be observed with autologous MSCs.

Second, and conversely, autologous MSCs might induce donor-specific hyporesponsiveness. There is precedent for such a postulate based on previous donor-specific transfusions data [24].

Third, the differentiation potential of MSCs could lead to the loss of the correct pattern of spatiotemporal development in a specific tissue or organ, with the formation of atypical cell types within it. Reports already exist of elevated levels of calcification in mice treated with MSCs to combat the effects of myocardial infarction [25].

Fourth, such differentiation and/or paracrine support for damaged tissue could lead to neoplasia. This has yet to be observed in practice, however, and the use of such cells in bone-marrow transplant without serious adverse consequences over the past 40 years is encouraging in this respect.

Fifth, the widespread dispersal of MSCs in vivo following infusion runs the risk of stimulating fibrosis through paracrine stimulation of tissue by MSC-secreted factors. Precedent for such a scenario exists. Recent clinical data from experiments using adipose-derived EPCs show immediate fibrosis following lipoinjection into adipose tissue [26].

Finally, given that MSCs have the capacity to modulate the immune system, the question of whether infusions of these cells will compromise overall immune surveillance arises. Initial primate studies have indicated that administration of high-dose allogeneic MSCs affects alloreactive immune responses [27].

Hemapoetic stem cells and transplantation

Pertinent to this is the recent substantial evidence showing induction of tolerance in combined bone-marrow and kidney transplantation for both HLA-matched and HLA-mismatched donor–recipient combinations [28]. Besides avoiding the need for immunosuppression, tolerance prevents ongoing chronic rejection, the most significant cause of graft loss. In order to achieve a state of donor-specific unresponsiveness, mixed lymphohematopoietic chimerism is of prime importance. This occurs when both host- and donor-derived hematopoietic progeny are observed in all blood lineages. Initial trials on HLA-matched combinations—performed more than 10 years ago—were on patients with multiple myeloma and end-stage renal failure who would not have been eligible for kidney transplantation [29]. Although the results quoted in the literature are promising, the technique is still in its infancy, with limited long-term follow-up [28,30], and is carried out by very few centers in the USA. The concept, however, provides a strong platform from which to emphasize the success of host tolerance induction and the complete withdrawal of immunosuppressive medication.

Pathfinder cells: an alternative to solid-organ pancreas transplantation?

A further cell type with potential for use in solid-organ transplantation has been described. This is a novel cell population, isolated from both adult rat and human tissues. These are termed pathfinder cells (PCs) [23,31], on the basis that they appear to navigate a path towards sites of damage in vivo. PCs have proven efficacy in regenerating tissue in a number of solid-organ damage models. Notably, these cells work across a species barrier, exert their influence on damaged tissue in a paracrine fashion, and have immunomodulatory properties. Their developmental point of origin remains to be defined.

These cells share many properties with MSCs, in that they can be isolated in culture with an adherent phenotype when grown on plastic and can form spherical cell clusters. They display paracrine interactions with immune cells that are already well documented for MSCs [32]. Unlike MSCs, these cells can be CD90, CD105, and CD73 negative.

Direct intravenous injection of rat or human PCs into streptozotocin (STZ)-induced diabetic mice resulted in a paracrine-mediated normalization of blood-glucose levels and restoration of mouse pancreatic architecture. Crucially, the insulin produced by these treated animals was principally mouse in origin and was of both type I (embryonic) and type II (adult) [23], indicative of stimulated developmental recapitulation. Notably, the PCs do not persist indefinitely after infusion—analogous to MSCs—and can only be detected at low levels ($<0.1\%$) 100 days after administration. These observations are also in keeping with previous reports suggesting a means for novel therapeutic intervention without making differentiated cells for transplantation ex vivo [31,33,34]. Significantly, PCs have demonstrated efficacy in rodent models of renal and cardiac ischemia, which bodes well for their development as a clinical cellular therapeutic.

Induced pluripotent stem cells

Derived as an alternative to working with stem cells, induced pluripotent stem (iPS) cells have been used to derive a number of specialized cell types and may eventually have a role in transplantation, though this would seem to be some way off at present. iPS derivation involves genetically manipulating adult cells to express a number of transcription factors normally required for maintaining stem cells in an undifferentiated state [35,36]. iPS cells show many similarities to ESCs in morphology, proliferation, and the capacity for teratoma formation. Tumor formation in chimeras following iPS-cell implantation precludes their use in transplantation. Recently, iPS cells have shown success when used to provide a model system for studying complex human disease conditions [37]. Such studies are an important correlate for the development of improved clinical strategies to treat disease. More recently, however, Pasi *et al.* have reported that iPS cells are genetically unstable and possess a range of abnormalities more associated with neoplastic transformation, which suggests a serious impediment to their use as a therapeutic cell source [38].

Neo-organogenesis for transplantation

Most current approaches, with the exception of PC therapy, use stem or progenitor cells to build tissue directly, rather than by way of induction of natural developmental pathways. Extensive work has allowed the definition of many stem-cell subtypes, several of which are pluripotent (as defined earlier), but persuading these cells to form the correct three-dimensional tissue architecture of mature organs has proven far more problematic.

All abdominal organs develop from a stem-cell population that aggregates, separates from surrounding structures (in the case of the kidney, with the formation of a tough connective tissue capsule), and induces a complex network of blood vessels, which allow growth to the large size of the mature organ. Further ingrowth of additional cell types, such as neuroendocrine pancreatic cells, may also be necessary before the mature organ is properly formed (Figure 7.1).

These steps lie between implantation of a stem-cell population and useful organ function, unless—as in the case of a bone-marrow or peripheral-blood stem-cell transplant—the desired function is one or more singly existing blood cell type. There is no better example of the difficulty of forming clinically useful tissue from stem-cell sources than the inability of the entire scientific world to develop something as conceptually simple as quality-controlled erythrocyte populations for transfusion, let alone a kidney.

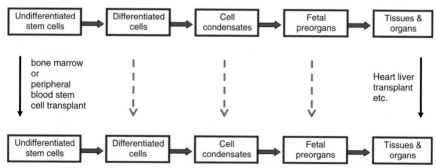

Figure 7.1 Schematic representation of the progress of organ development from undifferentiated stem-cell population to mature organ

Natural blueprints for stem cell–organ development: using fetal cells to grow an organ

Figure 7.2 shows that the fetal preorgan may be considered the natural blueprint for stem-cell assembly into the mature organ. Implantation of the fetal kidney rudiment has been described [39], but this cannot replicate the magnitude of glomerular filtration nor tubular function to sustain life [40,41]. Transplantation of the less well-defined pancreas rudiment has also shown promise, but it too remains some way from clinical practice [42].

Utilizing these fetal preorgans as a template to allow stem cells— microinjected into the preorgan before implantation—to form a functioning organ, has been attempted. In the case of the kidney, functioning human glomeruli and tubules have been demonstrated in preinjected rat fetal kidney grafts, but once again, this technology is some way short of being an alternative to kidney transplantation [43].

Creating tolerant adult organs

The fetal organ may only represent a blueprint for a small, immature organ, and may lack developmental cues relating to late prenatal and postnatal growth and development. The adult organ contains a fully formed connective-tissue architecture and vasculature and represents an alternative blueprint. Injection of autologous stem cells on to a decellularized human trachea has been successfully performed in a human patient [44], but this only requires a single epithelial layer to form on the inside of the decellularized platform. This is no more complex than the cells' behavior in culture. Nevertheless, it is a landmark for stem-cell transplantation.

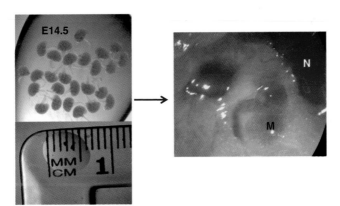

Figure 7.2 Experimental fetal-organ rudiment transplant. E14.5 rat fetal kidney preorgan, the metanephros (shown to scale). When transplanted to an adult rat abdomen, after 17 days the metanephros develops gross renal morphology (M) (next to native kidney (N) for scale). (Partially reproduced from (36) Clancy MJ, Marshall D, Dilworth M, Bottomley M, Ashton N, Brenchley P. Immunosuppression is essential for successful allogeneic transplantation of the metanephros. Transplantation 2009 July 27;88(2):151–9, with permission from Wolters Kluwer Health)

Repopulation of a heart with stem cells is also described experimentally [45], but the complexity of abdominal organs like the kidney, liver, and pancreas still remains a barrier to regrowing clinically useful and transplantable organs from stem-cell sources.

The future

Despite many remaining obstacles, the use of cellular therapies to augment the transplant team's armamentarium and to treat previously intractable conditions is exciting. Translation of these strategies is rapidly advancing, though a legion of unanswered questions remain with respect to both the basic biology and the long-term success of treatments. Will these therapies replace damaged tissue without addressing any underlying pathology? Will stem cells be differentiated in vitro to form solid organs for transplant, as they have with the relatively more simple trachea? What immune issues need to be dealt with? Except in bone-marrow transplantation, obtaining enough of a given cell type and ensuring the risk of cancer is minimized post-transplant also remain as barriers.

Despite these hurdles, cell therapies offer significant potential for treating previously intractable conditions and understanding the basic biological processes involved in development and tissue homeostasis. Progress since the hyperbolic promise of the first embryonic stem-cell lines seems to have been slow, but the next decade is likely to see cell-based treatments cement their clinical role.

References

1 Thomson JA, Itskovitz-Eldor J, Shapiro SS, Waknitz MA, Swiergiel JJ, Marshall VS, Jones JM. Embryonic stem cell lines derived from human blastocysts. *Science* 1998;282(5391):1145–1147.

2 Stevenson K, McGlynn L, Shiels PG. Stem cells: outstanding potential and outstanding questions. *Scott Med J* 2009;54(4):35–37.

3 Friedenstein AJ, Petrakova KV, Kurolesova AI, Frolova GP. Heterotopic of bone marrow. Analysis of precursor cells for osteogenic and hematopoietic tissues. *Transplantation* 1968;6:230–247.

4 Popp FC, Renner P, Eggenhofer E, Slowik P, Geissler EK, Piso P, Schlitt HJ, Dahlke MH. Mesenchymal stem cells as immunomodulators after liver transplantation. *Liver Transplantation* 2009;15(10):1192–1198.

5 Crop M, Baan C, Weimar W, Hoogduijn M. Potential of mesenchymal stem cells as immune therapy in solid-organ transplantation. *Transpl Int* 2009; 22(4):365–376.

6 Dominici M Le Blanc K, Mueller I, Slaper-Cortenbach I, Marini F, Krause D, Deans R, Keating A, Prockop DJ, Horwitz, E. Minimal criteria for defining multipotent mesenchymal stromal cells. *The International Society for Cellular Therapy position statement. Cytotherapy* 2006;8(4):315–317.

7 Frith JE, Thomson B, Genever P. Dynamic three-dimensional culture methods enhance mesenchymal stem cell properties and increase therapeutic potential. *Tissue Eng Part C Methods* 2010;16(4):735–749.

8 van Poll D, Parekkadan B, Cho CH, *et al.* Mesenchymal stem cell derived molecules directly modulate hepatocellular death and regenerationin vitro and in vivo. *Hepatology* 2008;47:1634–1638.

9 Imberti B, Morigi M, Tomasoni S, *et al*. Insulin-like growth factor-1 sustains stem cell mediated renal repair. *J Am Soc Nephrol* 2007;18:2921–2929.

10 Di Nicola M, Carlo-Stella C, Magni M, *et al*. Human bone marrow stromal cells suppress T-lymphocyte proliferation induced by cellular or nonspecific mitogenic stimuli. *Blood* 2002;99:3838.

11 Le Blanc K, Tammik L, Sundberg B, Haynesworth SE, Ringden O. Mesenchymal stem cells inhibit and stimulatemixed lymphocyte cultures and mitogenic responses independently of the major histocompatibility complex. *ScandJ Immunol* 2003;57:11.

12 Krampera M, Glennie S, Dyson J, *et al*. Bone marrow mesenchymal stem cells inhibit the response of naive and memory antigen-specific T cells to their cognate peptide. *Blood* 2003;101:3722.

13 Yeagy BA, Harrison F, Gubler MC, Koziol JA, Salomon DR, Cherqui S Kidney preservation by bone marrow cell transplantation in hereditary nephropathy. *Kidney Int* 2011;79(11):1198–1206.

14 Perico N, Casiraghi F, Introna M, Gotti E, Todeschini M, Cavinato RA, Capelli C, Rambaldi A, Cassis P, Rizzo P, Cortinovis M, Marasà M, Golay J, Noris M, Remuzzi G. Autologous mesenchymal stromal cells and kidney transplantation: a pilot study of safety and clinical feasibility. *Clin J Am Soc Nephrol* 2011;6(2):412–422.

15 Stevenson KS, McGlynn L, Hodge M, McLinden H, George WD, Davies RW, Shiels PG. Isolation, characterization, and differentiation of thy1.1-sorted pancreatic adult progenitor cell populations. *Stem Cells Dev* 2009;18(10): 1389–1398.

16 Diep CQ, Ma D, Deo RC, Holm TM, Naylor RW, Arora N, Wingert RA, Bollig F, Djordjevic G, Lichman B, Zhu H, Ikenaga T, Ono F, Englert C, Cowan CA, Hukriede NA, Handin RI, Davidson AJ. Identification of adult nephron progenitors capable of kidney regeneration in zebrafish. *Nature* 2011;470(7332):95–100.

17 Bilir BM, Guinette D, Karrer F, Kumpe DA, Krysl J, Stephens J, *et al*. Hepatocyte transplantation in acute liver failure. *Liver Transpl* 2000;6(1):32–40.

18 Schneider A, Attaran M, Meier PN, Strassburg C, Manns MP, Ott M, *et al*. Hepatocyte transplantation in an acute liver failure due to mushroom poisoning. *Transplantation* 2006;82(8):1115–1116.

19 Fisher RA, Strom SC. Human hepatocyte transplantation: worldwide results. *Transplantation* 2006;82(4):441–449.

20 Waelzlein JH, Puppi J, Dhawan A. Hepatocyte transplantation for correction of inborn errors of metabolism. *Curr Opin Nephrol Hypertens* 2009;18(6): 481–488.

21 Casiraghi F, Azzollini N, Cassis P, *et al*. Pre-transplant infusion of mesenchymal stem cells prolongs the survival of a semi-allogeneic heart transplant through the generation of regulatory T cells. *J Immunol* 2008;181:3933.

22 Popp FC, Eggenhofer E, Renner P, *et al*. Mesenchymal stem cells can induce long-term acceptance of solid organ allografts in synergy with low-dose mycophenolate. *Transpl Immunol* 2008;20:55.

23 Stevenson K, Chen D, McIntyre A, McGlynn L, Russell D, Montague P, Subramaniam M, George WD, Davies RW, Dorling A, Shiels PG. Complete reversal of streptozotocin induced diabetes by intravenous delivery of a novel adult rat cell type. *Rej Res* 2012 (in press).

24 Waanders MM, Roelen DL, Brand A, Claas FH. The putative mechanism of the immuno-modulating effect of HLA-DR shared allogeneic blood transfusions on the allo-immuneresponse. *Transfus Med Rev* 2005;19:281.

25 Breitbach M, Bostani T, Roell W, *et al*. Potential risks of bone marrow cell transplantation into infarcted hearts. *Blood* 2007;110:1362.

26 Yoshimura K, Aoi N, Suga H, *et al*. Ectopic fibrogenesis induced by transplantation of adipose-derived progenitor cell suspension immediately after lipoinjection. *Transplantation* 2008;85:1868.

27 Beggs KJ, Lyubimov A, Borneman JN, *et al*. Immunologic consequences of multiple, high-dose administration of allogeneic mesenchymal stem cells to baboons. *Cell Transplant* 2006;15:711.

28 Kawai T, Cosimi AB, Spitzer TR, Tolkoff-Rubin N, Suthanthiran M, Saidman SL, *et al*. HLA-mismatched renal transplantation without maintenance immunosuppression. *N Engl J Med* 2008;358(4):353–361.

29 Spitzer TR, Delmonico F, Tolkoff-Rubin N, McAfee S, Sackstein R, Saidman S, *et al*. Combined histocompatibility leukocyte antigen-matched donor bone marrow and renal transplantation for multiple myeloma with end stage renal disease: the induction of allograft tolerance through mixed lymphohematopoietic chimerism. *Transplantation* 1999;68(4):480–484.

30 Spitzer TR, Sykes M, Tolkoff-Rubin N, Kawai T, McAfee SL, Dey BR, *et al*. Long-term follow-up of recipients of combined human leukocyte antigen-matched bone marrow and kidney transplantation for multiple myeloma with end-stage renal disease. *Transplantation* 2011;91(6):672–676.

31 Shiels PG. Adult stem cells mitigate the effects of STZ diabetes.*Horizons in Medicine* 2004;17:241–249.

32 Yagi H, Soto-Gutierrez A, Parekkadan B, Kitagawa Y,Tompkins RG, Kobayashi N, Yarmush ML. Mesenchymalstem cells: mechanisms of immunomodulation and homing. *Cell Transplant* 2010;19:667–679.

33 Dor Y, Brown J, Martinez OI, Melton DA. Adult pancreatic beta-cells are formed by self-duplication rather than stem cell differentiation. *Nature* 2004;429:41–46.

34 Nir T, Melton DA, Dor Y. Recovery from diabetes in mice by beta cell regeneration. *J Clin Invest* 2007;117:2553–2561.

35 Meissner A, Wernig M, Jaenisch R. Direct reprogramming of genetically unmodified fibroblasts into pluripotent stem cells. *Nat Biotechnol* 2007;10:1177–1181.

36 Okita K, Ichisaka T, Yamanaka S. Generation of germline-competent induced pluripotent stem cells. *Nature* 2007; 448(7151):313–317.

37 Zhang J, Lian Q, Zhu G, Zhou F, Sui L, Tan C, Mutalif RA, Navasankari R, Zhang Y, Tse HF, Stewart CL, Colman A. A human iPSC model of Hutchinson Gilford Progeria reveals vascular smooth muscle and mesenchymal stem cell defects. *Cell Stem Cell* 2011;8(1):31–45.

38 Pasi CE, Dereli-Öz A, Negrini S, Friedli M, Fragola G, Lombardo A, Van Houwe G, Naldini L, Casola S, Testa G, Trono D, Pelicci PG, Halazonetis TD. Genomic instability in induced stem cells. *Cell Death Diff* 2011;18(5):745–753.

39 Hammerman MR. Transplantation of renal precursor cells: a new therapeutic approach. *Pediatr Nephrol* 2000;14(6):513–517.

40 Marshall D, Dilworth MR, Clancy M, Bravery CA, Ashton N. Increasing renal mass improves survival in anephric rats following metanephros transplantation. *Exp Physiol* 2007;92(1):263–271.

41 Clancy MJ, Marshall D, Dilworth M, Bottomley M, Ashton N, Brenchley P. Immunosuppression is essential for successful allogeneic transplantation of the metanephros. *Transplantation* 2009;88(2):151–159.

42 Hammerman MR. Xenotransplantation of embryonic pig kidney or pancreas to replace the function of mature organs. *J Transplant* 2011; doi:10.1155/2011/501749.

43 Yokoo T, Kawamura T. Xenobiotic kidney organogenesis: a new avenue for renal transplantation. *J Nephrol* 2009;22(3):312–317.
44 Baiguera S, Birchall MA, Macchiarini P. Tissue-engineered tracheal transplantation. *Transplantation* 2010;89(5):485–491.
45 Taylor DA. From stem cells and cadaveric matrix to engineered organs. *Curr Opin Biotechnol* 2009;20(5):598–605.

8 Intestinal Transplantation

Khalid M. Khan[1], Tun Jie[2], Chirag S. Desai[2], and Rainer W.G. Gruessner[2]

[1]Pediatric Liver & Intestine Transplant Program, University of Arizona, USA
[2]Department of Surgery, University of Arizona College of Medicine, USA

Introduction

Continuity with its environment makes the intestine a unique abdominal organ. Apart from its nutritional role, it contains a large amount of lymphoid tissue and intimately interacts with microbial flora. The lymphoid element within the gut has a necessary, complex immunological role, so it was always deemed an intuitive barrier to intestinal transplantation. Nevertheless, Richard Lillehei at the University of Minnesota saw the potential for transplanting the small intestine in patients with intestinal failure and performed the first such transplant in the 1960s [1]. Early refinements in surgical technique were followed by advances in immunosuppression and a better appreciation of post-transplant care; today, an intestinal transplant (ITx) is a well-established option in clinical practice.

Classification

The small intestine (jejunum to ileum) makes up the graft in an ITx. But in any particular recipient, the small intestine can be combined with the liver or with any of the abdominal viscera, including the abdominal wall if necessary (according to the "cluster" concept originally proposed by Starzl [2]). Therefore, the small intestine can be transplanted in isolation (an isolated intestinal transplant, or I-ITx), in combination with part or all of the liver (a liver–intestine transplant, or L-ITx), in combination with the stomach, liver, duodenum, and pancreas, all commonly transplanted en bloc, especially in small children (a multivisceral transplant, or MVTx), or in combination with the stomach, duodenum, and pancreas—excluding the liver (a modified MVTx). In addition, in certain recipients, the colon and/or part of the abdominal wall have been added. The use of living donors, though limited to specific centers in the USA, has been shown to be an effective option in ITx recipients.

Abdominal Organ Transplantation: State of the Art, First Edition.
Edited by Nizam Mamode and Raja Kandaswamy.
© 2013 Blackwell Publishing Ltd. Published 2013 by Blackwell Publishing Ltd.

Intestinal failure

The fundamental basis for an ITx is failure of the small intestine to maintain life with enteral intake. Short-bowel syndrome (SBS), a term often used synonymously with intestinal failure, refers to a malabsorptive state that results from an anatomical deficiency of the small intestine. SBS may also be functional in nature, where there is adequate length but poor function.

Etiology

In infants, intestinal failure is frequently caused by anatomical SBS. Most infants who undergo extensive resection of the small intestine now survive. The common congenital defects resulting in anatomical SBS are gastroschisis, intestinal atresia, and malrotation [3,4]. The improved survival of premature infants has resulted in a proportional increase in the number of infants whose SBS is due to resection for necrotizing enterocolitis. Other than anatomical SBS, intestinal failure is also caused by diffuse neuromuscular dysfunction, such as the total aganglionic form of Hirschsprung disease. In children and adults, a less frequent cause of intestinal failure is hollow visceral myopathy and neuropathy, resulting clinically in pseudo-obstruction. Diffuse mucosal disease (e.g. microvillus inclusion disease) is fatal without treatment; malabsorption can occur with polyposis [5].

In adults, the most common underlying cause of SBS is small-intestinal Crohn disease [6]. Other causes include a mesenteric vascular event such as arterial or venous thrombosis, arterial embolism, midgut volvulus, or other complications of surgery; extensive resection after trauma or after tumor removal; and radiation injury. Increasingly, complications after bariatric surgery, particularly after Roux-en-Y gastric-bypass procedures, are a cause of SBS [7].

Parenteral nutrition (PN) can be a lifesaving therapy for patients with intestinal failure. However, in PN patients, the liver may develop steatosis or cholestasis. In infants with SBS who are on chronic PN, cholestasis is more likely than steatosis. Liver disease is multifactorial and is associated with repeated sepsis; it may progress to liver failure. In children, clear progress in the management of SBS has occurred, so increasing numbers have been successfully weaned off PN. Surgical procedures to lengthen the small intestine have been developed, most notably the operation popularized by Bianchi [8] and the more recently described serial transverse enteroplasty (STEP) [9]. PN-related liver disease has been reversed by manipulating PN, specifically by lowering the amount of intravenous lipid infused daily and by changing to or adding a fish oil-based lipid preparation rich in omega-3 fatty acids [10].

A short segment of remaining small intestine, an absence of the ileocecal valve and colon, and severe dysmotility all are predictive of a poor outcome in patients with SBS; the level of the amino-acid citrulline has proven to be surrogate marker of small-intestinal function [11].

Prevalence

The exact prevalence of intestinal failure is unknown. Home PN Registry data, widely quoted, from 1992 show that about 40 000 patients required

PN each year at that time in the USA [12]. An Italian study estimated that 2.5 in every million children had intestinal failure [13]. Of course, the use of PN does not imply intestinal failure in every case, and most cases of SBS do not result in intestinal failure.

Recipient selection

An ITx is considered a rescue therapy with broad indications, as recognized by the US Centers for Medicare and Medicaid Services (CMS); these indications include development of progressive liver disease, loss of central-line access with thrombosis at two or more major line sites, recurrent episodes of dehydration despite intravenous therapy, and systemic fungal infection [7].

Ultimately, the need for an ITx will be determined by the individual patient's underlying intestinal pathology and size. Another key factor is whether or not a liver transplant is also required. For instance, in the case of pseudo-obstruction, repeated sepsis and loss of line sites are likely, so either an I-ITx or a modified MVTx may be necessary. Alternatively, in a small infant with SBS and progressive liver disease, the appropriate transplant is most likely an MVTx.

Clear contraindications to an ITx include systemic infection, preexisting severe neurological dysfunction, and the presence of malignancy. Severe cardiac dysfunction, whether acute or chronic, may also be a contraindication. Immune deficiency will present challenges. Age is not a usual limitation, but the overall health of the patient and their ability to tolerate an ITx are of importance. Patients with intestinal failure who live at home before being hospitalized for their transplant, as compared with inpatients, have a better outcome [7].

Evaluation of ITx candidates is based on similar protocols developed for other abdominal organ-transplant candidates and overlaps with protocols for liver-transplant candidates. In particular:

- In all ITx candidates, nutritional deficiency must be addressed.
- Detailed imaging of the intraabdominal vascular and enteric anatomy with computed tomography (CT) or magnetic resonance imaging (MRI) is a prerequisite, as is assessment for patency of central venous access sites.
- A liver biopsy and assessment for portal hypertension should be considered.
- ITx candidates with a history of vascular thrombosis should be evaluated for a procoagulant state.

Deceased-donor graft procurement

The overriding principle for graft selection is to obtain a match with the recipient, both immunologically and physically. In the prospective donor, a history of gastrointestinal disorders and abdominal operations should be fully evaluated. Before graft procurement, the donor's cardiovascular integrity, perfusion, and the degree of ischemia should be estimated. The presence of bowel sounds, documentation of a bowel movement, and the absence of blood in the stool are reassuring for intestinal integrity. Because most ITx recipients have a loss of abdominal domain due to prior surgeries, donors are usually selected whose weight is around 50–60% of the recipient's [14]. In most cases, vascular conduits are necessary; the need for them must be anticipated and agreed to with the other procurement teams preoperatively. The descending thoracic aorta, subclavian artery, and carotid artery may be useful when the iliac vessels are required by the liver and pancreatic procurement teams. Similarly, any pretreatment of the donor with Thymoglobulin, as is the practice in some centers, must be agreed to in advance with the other procurement teams.

The donor operation commences with a midline incision from the xiphisternum to the symphysis pubis. In general, the distal abdominal aorta is cannulated for flushing with University of Wisconsin (UW) solution. In I-ITx procurement, cannulation of the inferior mesenteric vein should be avoided, because it can cause graft edema due to outflow obstruction. The supraceliac aorta is encircled in preparation for crossclamping—taking care, in pediatric donors, to do so as proximally as possible, in order to use the descending thoracic aorta for necessary conduits.

I-ITx procurement

In the warm phase of I-ITx graft procurement, careful dissection is carried out at the base of the mesentery; the portal vein and superior mesenteric artery (SMA) are dissected just below the pancreatic uncinate process. Doing so makes it possible to use separately, from the same donor, both the pancreas and the small intestine. The small intestine is stapled just below the ligament of Treitz; distally, the colon is stapled at the level of the left branch of the middle colic vessel. If the pancreas is not to be procured as a separate graft for another recipient, I-ITx procurement is much easier. The SMA can be circled at its origin after a Catell maneuver and after a Kocher maneuver; then, after a cold flush, the pancreatic neck can be bisected and the intestine removed.

Procurement of other organs

After dissection of the vessels as already described, the tail of the pancreas and the spleen are mobilized from the retroperitoneum, taking care to avoid injury to the superior mesenteric vessels or to the inferior pancreaticoduo-denal arcade. The proximal duodenum is then dissected and divided at the level of the pylorus. A Carrel patch containing origins of the celiac trunk and SMA is taken with a wide margin, so that an aortic conduit can be used if required. The entire pancreas, spleen, small intestine, and liver are removed en bloc with an intact inferior vena cava (IVC) and duodenum. For an MVTx, the stomach is taken as well; for a modified MVTx, the liver is left.

The back-table procedure requires resection of the distal pancreas to the right of the mesenteric vessels, ligating the branches draining the uncinate process and oversewing the pancreatic remnant. A more recent trend is to transplant the entire pancreas. The left gastric artery and splenic arteries must be ligated. The gastroduodenal and inferior pancreaticoduodenal arteries are preserved. For all grafts, heparin is administered, the distal aorta is ligated and cannulated, the graft is flushed with UW solution, and ice is used for cooling.

Deceased-donor recipient operation

The recipient operation may present a challenge as a result of underlying disorders. SBS is associated with prior multiple procedures and, therefore, intraabdominal adhesions. The abdominal domain may be limited, especially if part of the small intestine is congenitally absent. Major venous access sites may be reduced from sepsis and thrombosis. Anticoagulation needs must be anticipated.

I-ITx recipient operation
Usually, a midline incision is made. If possible, the superior mesenteric vein (SMV) and SMA are dissected at the base of the mesentery; with or without conduits, the graft SMA and SMV are anastomosed. Then proximal small-intestinal continuity is established with an end-to-side or side-to-side anastomosis. Distally, either an end-ileal stoma ("chimney") or a loop ileostomy is created; distal intestinal continuity is established either end-to-end or side-to-end with the colon. In many cases, the mesentery is scarred, and primary portal drainage is not possible, so the intestine is drained centrally; the SMV is anastomosed to the IVC. Similarly, the SMA may be anastomosed to the infrarenal aorta with the addition of a conduit.

L-ITx recipient operation
A midline incision is made, with bilateral subcostal extensions. Dissection of the liver hilum allows the hepatic artery and common bile duct to be ligated. The portal vein is skeletonized and the infrahepatic IVC is isolated, for construction of a portocaval shunt. Then the liver is dissected from the cava, as for piggyback liver transplants. The infrarenal aorta is exposed for anastomosis. An aortic donor conduit is then placed on the infrarenal aorta to facilitate inflow to the graft; in some cases, a supraceliac aorta is used. The hepatic veins are clamped and the liver removed. An end-to-side portocaval shunt is constructed. The graft is brought into the field, and a suprahepatic caval anastomosis is performed in a piggyback fashion. In children, the entire aorta with the origin of the celiac trunk and the SMA is used for inflow. In adults, an iliac-Y-graft can be used to establish inflow. Enteral continuity is reestablished with a side-to-side duodenoduodenostomy or jejunojejunostomy. The distal anastomosis is made as for an I-ITx recipient operation. All L-ITx recipients undergo gastrojejunostomy tube placement for postoperative tube feeding.

MVTx recipient operation

The recipient's entire splanchnic circulation is removed, along with associated viscera; the pancreas, the spleen, the root of the intestinal mesentery, the stomach, and the liver are all removed together. The celiac trunk and SMA are ligated, preserving the IVC for piggyback allograft transplants. Vascular anastomoses and enteral continuity are reestablished, as for L-ITx grafting. Due to the high incidence of gastric stasis, a pyloroplasty is also performed.

For small pediatric recipients, size-matched organs may not be available [15]. Using a larger deceased donor is often the most workable option; under those circumstances, alternatives for abdominal closure include abdominal expansion using nonbiological or biological mesh, acellular dermal matrix, human skin, a rotational flap, and/or a donor abdominal wall graft implanted into the recipient's iliac or epigastric vessels [16–19]. In some MVTx recipients, the donor's colon and spleen have been included—the spleen for technical reasons, namely the potential of splenic function and better immune tolerance [20]. Including the spleen has been shown to reduce intestinal graft rejection and to increase the recipient's response to pneumococcal vaccination, without an increase in the incidence of post-transplant lymphoproliferative disease (PTLD) or of graft-versus-host disease (GVHD) [21].

The previous standard was to use organs from deceased but heart-beating donors. The donor pool has now been expanded by successfully using deceased donors who have previously undergone resuscitation, whose blood group did not match the recipient's, who had a positive T-cell crossmatch result, and who were positive for cytomegalovirus (CMV), even if their recipient was negative [22].

Living donors

The concept of using a living donor in an ITx is an extension of the practice of using living donors in other types of solid-organ transplant. The ability to resect and reanastomose the small intestine has long been a natural part of the surgeon's repertoire; procuring part of the small intestine from a healthy living donor was an intuitive next step. The first successful living-donor ITx was performed in Germany (1988) by Deltz *et al.*, using immunosuppression based on cyclosporine A (CyA) [23]. As known from other solid-organ transplants, the use of living donors has advantages, such as human leukocyte antigen (HLA) matching—as exemplified in successful transplants between identical twins [24–26]—shorter graft ischemia time, a positive impact on waiting-list mortality, and the ability to perform the transplant electively.

The potential risk for the living donor is always a concern. The size of the intestinal graft that could be procured from ITx living donors was an issue until Gruessner developed a standardized technique in 1997 at the University of Minnesota [27]. This technique entails using 120–150 cm of the distal jejunum and ileum. The ileocecal valve and a 20 cm segment of the distal ileum are preserved in the living donor, in order to assure normal absorptive sufficiency after donation [28].

Living-donor selection

Common practices from other types of solid-organ transplant have been adapted for living-donor selection. Broadly, they can be categorized as relating to immunological matching (e.g. ABO, HLA, lymphocyte crossmatching); assessment of comorbidities and body habitus (e.g. cardiovascular, psychosocial, anesthesia, medication, and allergy status, as well as laboratory testing for infectious diseases, chemistry profiles, kidney function, liver disease, and hematological and nutritional sufficiency); and anatomical considerations (e.g. concerning any prior surgeries and particularly the blood supply to the small intestine). A CT-angiogram with three-dimensional reconstruction can be said to be the standard imaging modality, with particular attention given to the dimensions of the proposed arterial supply; selective mesenteric angiography is typically restricted for equivocal prospective living donors [29]. The explanation of risks to prospective living donors should include specifically the possibility of diarrhea, malabsorption, and intestinal obstruction.

Living-donor operation

The operation in living donors largely remains the same as described by Gruessner. A lower midline incision is made to present the small intestine, which is then measured from the ligament of Treitz to the ileocecal valve; a length of ileum/jejunum is removed, as already noted (Figure 8.1). Drains are not used. The typical hospital stay is less than a week. Return to work is usually within 3 weeks after donation, with limitations on lifting weight for up to 6 weeks.

Living-donor recipient operation

The ITx operation in living-donor recipients is similar to that in deceased-donor recipients. The salient issues involve vascular attachments to the infrarenal aorta and vena cava (Figure 8.2). The first living-donor L-ITx recipient was a sensitized 2-year-old who underwent a sequential transplant. First, the left lateral segment of the liver from the mother was used, followed by the ileal graft (also from the mother) a week later. The outcome was described as good for both the child and the mother [30]. The advantage of the sequential L-ITx technique is that it allows time for recipient desensitization.

Post-transplant care

The important issues in the early post-transplant period include meticulous attention to fluid balance, close surveillance for arterial vascular compromise with frequent examination of the stoma, and Doppler evaluation of hepatic

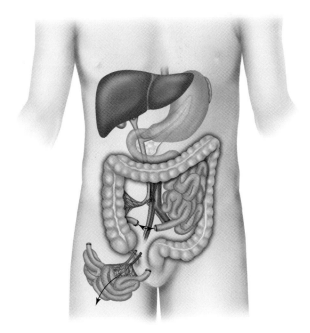

Figure 8.1 Living-donor operation for an isolated intestinal transplant (I-ITx): about 120–150 cm of small intestine is removed, preserving 20 cm of distal-most ileum

vessels. Serial small-intestinal biopsies through the distal stoma are necessary to diagnose early rejection. Secretory diarrhea can be caused by acute cellular rejection (ACR) or viral infection, most notably CMV. Enteral feeding is started with an elemental formula and advanced gradually.

Immunosuppression and rejection

Induction therapy (with interleukin (IL)-2 receptor blockade and/or antithymocyte globulin) has resulted in improved graft and patient survival rates in the first year post-transplant; induction agents are now included in some combination in most regimens, along with steroids [31]. Tacrolimus is standard for maintenance immunosuppression. Some institutions include mycofenolate mofetil in the initial months post-transplant; sirolimus has also been used [32]. Notably, alemtuzumab use has been reduced in children because of side effects [33].

In ITx recipients, ACR occurs more frequently, and is more severe, than rejection of any other abdominal organ [33]. Historically, two-thirds of ITx recipients experienced ACR [34]; with newer regimens, only one-third of ITx and MVTx recipients now experience it [7]. Graft loss occurs from severe intractable ACR and chronic allograft dysfunction, which is

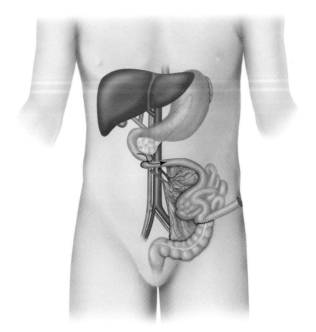

Figure 8.2 Isolated intestinal transplant (I-ITx): the proximal end of the graft is anastomosed side to side; distally, an end ileostomy is created with an anastomosis of the distal part of the graft and native colon just proximal to the stoma

pathologically described as a vascular event. Subclinical rejection (SCR) has been described [35], while acute vascular rejection (AVR) is not well defined [36]. Anti-inflammatory monoclonal antibodies against tumor necrosis factor (TNF)-α have been shown to be effective in treating ACR and may be useful for treating chronic enteropathy [37], with results similar to those with alemtuzumab [38]. Ultimately, chronic graft loss due to vascular changes cannot be adequately treated and is responsible for the poor long-term outcome in most ITx recipients. A recent finding is that mutations in the gene coding for nucleotide-binding oligomerization domain-containing protein 2 (NOD2)—that are typically associated with Crohn disease—may have a role in rejection [39].

Post-transplant immunosuppression in living-donor and deceased-donor ITx recipients is broadly similar. The Chicago group has reported a low incidence of bacterial infection post-transplant in their living-donor recipients, but the true impact on living-donor recipients of a short cold-ischemia time and of genetic matching has yet to be realized, especially when balanced against greater vascular challenges and limited graft length; nonetheless, the results, in general, of living-donor and deceased-donor transplants are comparable, as evidenced by scrutiny of data from the United Network for Organ Sharing (UNOS).

Patient and graft outcome

The most recent estimates suggest a survival rate of 90% in ITx recipients in centers with the greatest experience [7]. The long-term graft survival rate has remained about 60%; the rate abruptly worsens in pediatric patients after 3 years post-transplant [40]. Early deaths are mainly caused by sepsis (40–50%) and rejection (10%) [41]. Later deaths are also frequently caused by sepsis and rejection, along with PTLD (6–8%, with a peak incidence at 2 years post-transplant) [42]. The outcome of PTLD has improved with rituximab [43].

Cost and quality of life

A poor quality of life with associated neuropsychological complications is typical of patients with intestinal failure on PN. A recent review noted that, because of the limited number of studies and the preliminary nature of findings, strong conclusions cannot yet be drawn regarding quality of life in ITx recipients; however, the data so far were judged as encouraging. The cost of a transplant involving the small intestine has been examined in North America and Europe and is roughly similar on both continents. An ITx may be cost-effective as early as 2 years post-transplant, as compared with continued PN [44].

Summary and future directions

An ITx can be offered to patients with intestinal failure who are facing possible death from recurrent septicemia, from central-line loss, and/or from liver failure. For patients on PN with a pseudo-obstruction or intractable enteropathy, the mortality rate is high, so they should be considered for an ITx at an early stage of their disease. Living-donor transplants are not yet widespread. Future directions in this field may involve a reduction in the number of potential ITx recipients, thanks to hoped-for advances in the care of patients with intestinal failure; advances in immunosuppression for ITx recipients; elucidation of the mechanism of chronic graft loss; and strides in tissue engineering.

References

1 Lillehei RC, Idezuki Y, Feemster JA, *et al.* Transplantation of stomach, intestine, and pancreas: experimental and clinical observations. *Surgery* 1967;62(4):721–741.

2 Starzl TE, Todo S, Tzakis A, *et al.* The many faces of multivisceral transplantation. *Surg Gynecol Obstet* 1991;172:335–344.

3 Duro D, Kamin D, Duggan C. Overview of pediatric short bowel syndrome. *J Pediatr Gastroenterol Nutr* 2008;47(Suppl 1):S33–S36.

4 Spencer AU, Neaga A, West B, *et al.* Pediatric short bowel syndrome: redefining predictors of success. *Ann Surg* 2005;242:403–408.

5 Grant D, Abu-Elmagd K, Reyes J, *et al.*; Intestine Transplant Registry. 2003 report of the intestine transplant registry: a new era has dawned. *Ann Surg* 2005;241(4):607–613.

6 Raman M, Gramlich L, Whittaker S, Allard JP. Canadian home total parenteral nutrition registry: preliminary data on the patient population. *Can J Gastroenterol* 2007;21(10):643–648.

7 Fishbein TM. Intestinal transplantation. *N Engl J Med* 2009;361:998–1008.

8 Bianchi A. Intestinal loop lengthening: a technique for increasing small intestinal length. *J Pediatr Surg* 1980;15:145–151.

9 Kim HB, Fauza D, Garza J, *et al.* Serial transverse enteroplasty (STEP): a novel bowel lengthening procedure. *J Pediatr Surg* 2003;38:425–429.

10 Diamond IR, Sterescu A, Pencharz PB, Kim JH, Wales PW. Changing the paradigm: Omegaven for the treatment of liver failure in pediatric short bowel syndrome. *J Pediatr Gastroenterol Nutr* 2009;48(2):209–215.

11 Crenn P, Messing B, Cynober L. Citrulline as a biomarker of intestinal failure due to enterocyte mass reduction. *Clin Nutr* 2008;27(3):328–339.

12 Buchman AL. Etiology and initial management of short bowel syndrome. *Gastroenterology* 2006;130(2 Suppl 1):S5–S15.

13 Guarino A, De Marco G; Italian National Network for Pediatric Intestinal Failure. Natural history of intestinal failure, investigated through a national network-based approach. *J Pediatr Gastroenterol Nutr* 2003;37(2):136–141.

14 Tzakis A, Kato T, Levy D, *et al.* 100 multivisceral transplants at a single center. *Ann Surg* 2005;242:480–490.

15 Carlsen B, Farmer D, Busuttil R, *et al.* Incidence and management of abdominal wall defects after intestinal and multivisceral transplantation. *Plast Reconstr Surg* 2007;119:1247–1255.

16 de Ville de Goyet J, Mitchell A, Mayer AD, *et al.* En block combined reduced-liver and small bowel transplants: from large donors to small children. *Transplantation* 2000;69:555–559.

17 DiBenedetto F, Lauro A, Masetti M, *et al.* Use of prosthetic mesh in difficult abdominal wall closure after small bowel transplantation. *Transplant Proc* 2005;37:2272–2274.

18 Asham E, Uknis ME, Rastellini C, *et al.* Acellular dermal matrix provides a good option for abdominal wall closure following small bowel transplantation: a case report. *Transplant Proc* 2006;38:1770–1771.

19 Levi AG, Tzakis AG, Kato T, *et al.* Transplantation of the abdominal wall. *Lancet* 2003;361:2173–2176.

20 Stepkowski S, Bitter-Suermann H, Duncan W. Evidence supporting an in vivo role of T suppressor cells in spleen allograft induced tolerance. *Transplant Proc* 1986;18:207.

21 Kato T, Tzakis A, Selvaggi G, *et al.* Transplantation of the spleen. *Effect of splenic allograft in human multivisceral transplantation. Ann Surg* 2007;246: 436–446.

22 Gondolesi G, Fauda M. Technical refinements in small bowel transplantation. *Curr Opin Organ Transplant* 2008;13(3):259–265.

23 Deltz E, Mengel W, Hamelmann H. Small bowel transplantation: report of a clinical case. *Prog Pediatr Surg* 1990;25:90–96.

24 Morris JA, Johnson DL, Rimmer JA, *et al*. Identical-twin small-bowel transplant for desmoid tumour. *Lancet* 1995;345(8964):1577–1578.

25 Calne RY, Friend PJ, Middleton S, *et al*. Intestinal transplant between two of identical triplets. *Lancet* 1997;350(9084):1077–1078.

26 Morel P, Kadry Z, Charbonnet P, Bednarkiewicz M, Faidutti B. Paediatric living related intestinal transplantation between two monozygotic twins: a 1-year follow-up. *Lancet* 2000;355(9205):723–724.

27 Gruessner R, Sharp H. Living related intestinal transplantation: first report of a standardized surgical technique. *Transplantation* 1997;11:271–274.

28 Testa G, Panaro F, Schena S, *et al*. Living related small bowel transplantation: donor surgical technique. *Ann Surg* 2004;240:779–784.

29 Panaro F, Testa G, Balakrishnan N, *et al*. Living related small bowel transplantation in children: 3-dimensional computed tomography donor evaluation. *Pediatr Transplant* 2004;8(1):65–70.

30 Testa G, Holterman M, John E, *et al*. Combined living donor liver/small bowel transplantation. *Transplantation* 2005;79:1401–1404.

31 Vianna RM, Mangus RS, Fridell JA, *et al*. Induction immunosuppression with Thymoglobulin and rituximab in intestinal and multivisceral transplantation. *Transplantation* 2008;85:1290–1293.

32 Fishbein TM, Florman S, Gondolesi G, *et al*. Intestinal transplantation before and after the introduction of sirolimus. *Transplantation* 2002;73:1538–1542.

33 Garcia M, Delacruz V, Ortiz R, *et al*. Acute cellular rejection grading scheme for human gastric allografts. *Hum Pathol* 2004;35:343.

34 Selvaggi G, Gaynor JJ, Moon J, *et al*. Analysis of acute cellular rejection episodes in recipients of primary intestinal transplantation: a single-center, 11-year experience. *Am J Transplant* 2007;7:1249.

35 Takahashi H, Kato T, Selvaggi G, *et al*. Subclinical rejection in the initial postoperative period in small intestinal transplantation: a negative influence on graft survival. *Transplantation* 2007;84:689.

36 Ruiz P, Garcia M, Pappas P, *et al*. Mucosal vascular alterations in isolated small-bowel allografts: relationship to humoral sensitization. *Am J Transplant* 2003;3:43.

37 Pascher A, Radke C, Dignass A, *et al*. Successful infliximab treatment of steroid and OKT3 refractory acute cellular rejection in two patients after intestinal transplantation. *Transplantation* 2003;76:615.

38 Tzakis AG, Kato T, Nishida S, *et al*. Alemtuzumab (Campath-1H) combined with tacrolimus in intestinal and multivisceral transplantation. *Transplantation* 2003;75:1512.

39 Fishbein T, Novitskiy G, Mishra L, *et al*. NOD2-expressing bone marrow-derived cells appear to regulate epithelial innate immunity of the transplanted human small intestine. *Gut* 2008;57(3):323–330.

40 Ruiz P, Kato T, Tzakis A. Current status of transplantation of the small intestine. *Transplantation* 2007;83:1–6.

41 Grant D, Abu-Elmagd K, Reyes J, *et al*. On behalf of the Intestine Transplant Registry 2003 report of the intestine transplant registry: a new era has dawned. *Ann Surg* 2005;241:607.

42 Ruiz P, Soares MF, Garcia M, *et al*. Lymphoplasmacytic hyperplasia (possible pre-PTLD) has varied expression and appearance in intestinal transplant recipients receiving Campath immunosuppression. *Transplant Proc* 2004;36:386.

43 Nishida S, Kato T, Burney T, *et al*. Rituximab treatment for posttransplantation lymphoproliferative disorder after small bowel transplantation. *Transplant Proc* 2002;34:957.

44 Sudan D. Cost and quality of life after intestinal transplantation. *Gastroenterology* 2006;130(2 Suppl 1):S158.

9 Pediatric Renal Transplantation

Stephen D. Marks

Department of Paediatric Nephrology, Great Ormond Street Hospital
for Children NHS Trust, UK

Introduction

The long-term outcomes for children with end-stage renal failure (ESRF)
have improved over the last few decades with the development of specialist pediatric nephrology and renal-transplantation services throughout
the world. This requires a dedicated multidisciplinary team of pediatric
nephrologists, as well as general and other subspecialist pediatricians,
pediatric renal-transplantation, urological, and general surgeons, specialist
nurses, pharmacists, and dietitians, plus additional allied-health professionals and psychosocial team members. In the past, when children were
born anuric in nonobstructive ESRF, the only medical option was to offer
symptom-care therapy and allow the child to die. Nowadays, if the neonatal
course is uneventful with good cardiorespiratory status, dialysis can be
offered as a bridge to renal transplantation in the second year of life (and in
some circumstances, earlier). If a child has a good functioning renal allograft with minimal complications, this can give an excellent quality of life.
However, it is not always possible to predict which children are going to do
well, with good physical, psychological, growth, and pubertal development.

The intensive management of children with ESRF is complex and practice
varies around the world. The causes of ESRF are different and the long-
term outcome, with multiple transplantations in the future, has to be
considered. This chapter will focus on the differences between children
and adults with respect to the causes of ESRF, pretransplantation work-
up, peritransplantation management, and the subsequent course after
transplantation.

Pediatric ESRF

One of the most powerful moments in an adult's life is seeing their unborn
child for the first time on an ultrasound. This potentially joyous occasion
can be devastating for parents if there is evidence of significant fetal

Abdominal Organ Transplantation: State of the Art, First Edition.
Edited by Nizam Mamode and Raja Kandaswamy.
© 2013 Blackwell Publishing Ltd. Published 2013 by Blackwell Publishing Ltd.

renal disease. Antenatal ultrasound screening has completely transformed perinatal nephro-urological practice through identification of fetuses with significant renal abnormalities who may be born with severe kidney and/or respiratory failure [1]. However, practice varies throughout the world, with routine antenatal ultrasound scanning occurring at various times throughout the pregnancy, but usually at least at 20-weeks' gestation, when most abnormalities will be identified. In addition, many units in the UK offer early scanning at 12-weeks' gestation, with some countries also offering routine third-trimester ultrasound scanning. Antenatal ultrasound can identify other severe organ abnormalities, allowing a discussion of potential severe comorbidities associated with poorer prognosis. This allows time to counsel parents in the options, which may include termination, antenatal intervention (such as vesicoamniotic shunting), and planned intervention (such as being born in a unit with a link to pediatric nephrological center). However, despite antenatal ultrasound screening, some cases of renal abnormality are missed until a child presents with symptoms and/or signs of chronic kidney disease (CKD) or ESRF. Some cases, such as congenital nephrotic syndrome, may have no detected abnormalities until birth (although they may be diagnosed antenatally by elevated maternal alfafetoprotein levels and/or via a previous affected child by prenatal genetic diagnosis). There may be a delay in diagnosis until the neonate or infant presents with massive proteinuria, hypoalbuminemia, and resultant edema.

The causes of childhood ESRF differ from those in adults, who usually have diabetes mellitus, hypertension, or glomerular disease. The commonest cause of CKD and ESRF is congenital abnormalities of the kidneys and urinary tract (CAKUT; Figure 9.1). This usually manifests as congenitally malformed kidneys with bilateral renal dysplasia, which may be associated with vesico-ureteric reflux and/or obstructive uropathy—namely posterior urethral valves in boys. There needs to be full urological and

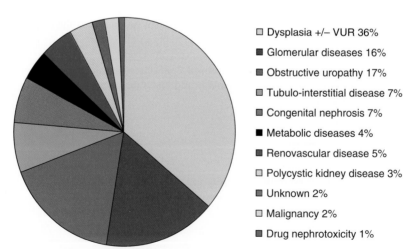

□ Dysplasia +/– VUR 36%
■ Glomerular diseases 16%
■ Obstructive uropathy 17%
□ Tubulo-interstitial disease 7%
■ Congenital nephrosis 7%
■ Metabolic diseases 4%
■ Renovascular disease 5%
□ Polycystic kidney disease 3%
■ Unknown 2%
□ Malignancy 2%
■ Drug nephrotoxicity 1%

Figure 9.1 Causes of ESRF in childhood. Data from the 11th annual United Kingdom Renal Registry pediatric end-stage renal failure report [2]

transplant-surgical consideration for pretransplant assessment in this group of patients [3]. Many cases of CAKUT will be caused by known genetic mutations, but at present these only account for 15% of cases in cohorts of nonsyndromic patients with renal hypodysplasia [4]. Children with congenital abnormalities may present with ESRF at any age, from antenatally to birth to adolescence. The most common genetic cause of ESRF within the first 2 decades of life is one of the hereditary cystic renal diseases, called juvenile nephronophthisis [5].

There is increased glomerular disease in children with ESRF, with the commonest cause being steroid-resistant nephrotic syndrome secondary to the histopathological diagnosis of primary focal and segmental glomerulosclerosis; this may also be resistant to other immunosuppressive drugs and has a 30–50% chance of recurring in the renal allograft. All children should have full genetic studies before embarking on renal transplantation, in order to try and evaluate the risk of recurrence post-transplantation, which may impact on the decision regarding identification of possible living related or deceased donors.

Over the last decade, increasing consideration has been given to children with ESRF who also have multisystem and metabolic conditions, some of whom have multiorgan transplant requirements. Options include simultaneous pancreas and kidney transplantation (usually for adults with type-I insulin-dependent diabetes mellitus, but also considered for children with hemolytic uremic syndrome who develop insulin-dependent diabetes mellitus) and possibly combined or sequential liver–kidney transplantation for primary hyperoxaluria type 1 [6]. There is also an increasing epidemic of CKD and ESRF caused by calcineurin nephrotoxicity from other solid-organ transplantation, such as cardiac, lung, and lung–cardiac transplantation [7].

Pretransplantation work-up

The patient and renal allograft survival rate for children receiving renal transplantation for ESRF has improved over the last decade and is comparable to that in adults (Figure 9.2). The pretransplantation work-up requires a multidisciplinary-team approach, involving physicians (pediatricians, pediatric nephrologists, and other subspecialists; anesthetists; intensivists), surgeons (pediatric surgeons; urologists; transplant surgeons) and specialized nurses, pharmacists, dietitians, psychologists, and other members of the psychosocial team.

Most pediatric renal-transplantation centers state a minimum weight of 10 kg before transplantation (but that excludes consideration of fluid status and the possible increased weight of native organs, and in fact length (which would give an indication of the intra-abdominal vessel size) would be more appropriate).

The views of pediatric renal-transplantation units around the world vary, but most aim for the gold standard of preemptive living related renal transplantation where possible [8]—with the closest immunological match—as the focus is on quality and quantity of life. It is important to

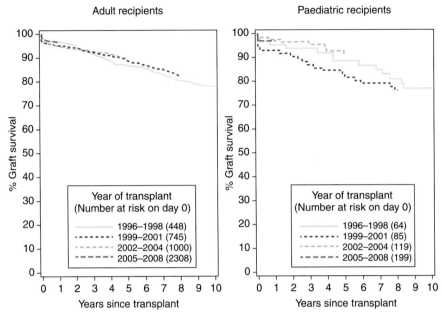

Figure 9.2 Ten-year renal allograft survival from first living-donor renal transplantation in adult and pediatric recipients in the UK. (Data supplied and reproduced with permission from National Health Service Blood and Transplant (NHSBT))

note that children will probably require multiple renal transplants during their lifetime. Some units wait for the requirement for dialysis before listing for deceased-donor renal transplants and exclude mismatched parental antigens (which can avoid subsequent sensitization), keeping the option of living related transplantation for the second renal transplant. However, the best long-term outcomes are for transplantation as opposed to dialysis, and living-donor renal-transplantation outcomes are better than outcomes from deceased donors, particularly when dialysis can be avoided [8].

The aim of the pretransplantation work-up is to try and plan for the best outcome for the prospective renal-transplant recipient, with individualized care according to risk stratification. This allows time for full vaccination, ensuring that all patients have immunity to potential preventable infectious complications before being transplanted. All prospective pediatric renal-transplant recipients should have the routine vaccination schedule (including diphtheria, tetanus, pertussis, polio, hemophilus influenzae, meningococcal, pneumococcal, measles, mumps, and rubella), BCG vaccination (Mantoux testing first in older children), hepatitis B (when hepatitis B surface-antigen-negative), varicella (when varicella immunoglobulin G (IgG)-negative), and repeat measles vaccination (where measles IgG-negative).

Pediatric recipients are at increased risk of early renal-allograft thrombosis due to lower renal perfusion pressures, especially small children, and a full prothrombotic screening should be undertaken if there is a personal and family history of thrombosis; anticoagulation policies should be adapted according to the results. All patients require cardiological assessment (with electrocardiography and echocardiography) as well as bladder, renal, and abdominal-vessel ultrasound screening. Patients with hostile bladders require full bladder function and urological assessment, which will typically involve urodynamic assessment of flow rate, volumes, and emptying [3]. A number of options are available to ensure that the bladder is safe for transplantation, including urinary diversion, a drainage procedure such as a Mitrofanoff, and bladder augmentation. There are currently no clearly accepted urodynamic criteria for intervention, and few studies have been performed. Combined management of these children in centers with adequate urological and transplant expertise is essential; if the bladder does not empty adequately, drainage will be required, and a small, poorly compliant bladder will probably require augmentation. The timing of such procedures in relation to transplantation is also uncertain, although there is some evidence that simultaneous transplantation and bladder surgery may lead to more complications [3]. Patients with abnormal or uncertain abdominal-vessel ultrasound screening should have magnetic resonance venography (MRV) performed [9]. Patients with increased risk of developing new-onset diabetes after transplantation (NODAT) (such as those with cystinosis) require full assessment. All patients require pretransplantation assessment by a pediatric transplantation physician, surgeon, and anesthetist.

Living-donor renal transplantation

Living-donor renal transplantation can be performed as a planned event when both donor and recipient are known to be healthy. It has improved patient and renal allograft survival, with reduced morbidity and acute rejection rates. However, there is a donor morbidity and mortality risk of 15 and 0.03%, respectively—with shorter hospital stay and less postoperative pain—after laparoscopic donation, which is now routine in most centers. There are additional aspects to consider with respect to pediatric renal transplantation when embarking on identification of possible living donors (who are usually the parents), as implantation of an adult organ into a pediatric recipient is more challenging. It may require surgery (for donor and recipient) in different hospitals, so safe and efficient transfer of organs to reduce cold-ischemia time is essential. Early postoperative communication must be available between donor and recipient. In our practice, we have used an Internet video link to facilitate this, although most of our donors are able to visit their respective recipients (in different hospitals) on the third postoperative day after laparoscopic donation. Unfortunately, around 20% of parents find they are unable to be donors due to identification of medical problems (including detection of unknown illnesses, abnormal kidneys, and solitary kidney), psychological or social issues which preclude donation, or other barriers (such as ABO incompatibility or preformed anti-human leukocyte antigen (HLA) antibodies), which may be overcome. As in adults with ESRF, unrelated donors can be considered, but improved long-term outcomes are related to minimizing HLA mismatching and subsequent sensitization, as children are likely to require retransplantation during their lifetime. Therefore, ABO-incompatible transplantation [10–13] and paired-exchange schemes should be considered for some pediatric recipients, where no living related donor is suitable.

Families should be counseled regarding the fact that children are at a higher risk of developing post-transplant lymphoproliferative disease (PTLD) due to being Epstein–Barr-virus (EBV)-naïve, while most adult donors are EBV-positive (so many children are transplanted with EBV mismatch).

In the UK, after both donor and recipient have completed their medical and psychosocial pretransplantation work-ups, the Human Tissue Authority undertakes independent assessments of all donor–recipient pairs to check suitability.

Deceased-donor renal transplantation

Most organ-donation systems give priority to children. In the UK, patients who are on-call and listed for deceased-donor renal transplantation prior to their 18th birthday have priority for receiving organs through the national scheme of National Health Service Blood and Transplant (NHSBT). This highlights the transplantation community's acknowledgement of the multiple reasons for prioritizing children and adolescents for renal transplantation, due to their life expectancy and lifelong requirement for ESRF management, as well as specific pediatric issues with respect to physical and psychosocial aspects of education, family life (including effect on siblings), and physical and psychological growth and development. The life expectancy is almost doubled if a child reaches the age of 18 with a functioning transplant—as opposed to being on dialysis [14]—with improved development and growth potential (including increased final adult height with a functioning renal allograft). This equates to a two-thirds reduced mortality rate in transplanted children compared to those on dialysis, as increased mortality is a function of the dialysis treatment itself [15,16]

The increased pediatric morbidity and mortality rates associated with hemodialysis are related to the inherent difficulties of venous-line and arteriovenous-fistulae formation, which produce higher risks of access loss. There is also an increased risk of infectious complications—with peritonitis and failing peritoneum—in children on peritoneal dialysis. The thrombotic rate of the major intra-abdominal vessels is increased in children requiring dialysis from birth, which may reduce vascular access for transplantation. Practical issues include potentially reduced educational attainment, as a result of time off school due to ill health, and in-center hemodialysis constraints, especially with increased travel to pediatric units due to the limited number of specialized centers.

Most units consider utilizing organs from deceased donors aged from 5 to 55 years. Pediatric donors under 5 years of age lead to an increased risk of renal-allograft thrombosis and other technical problems in pediatric recipients, so they are no longer routinely used in the UK, but they may be considered for use en bloc [17,18]. To improve the donor pool, consideration should be given to the use of organs from non-heart-beating deceased donors.

There may be contraindications to the use of kidneys from deceased donors with several adverse factors ("marginal donors") in pediatric recipients. These include donors with malignancy (such as primary brain malignancy or recent treatment of malignancy), infection (death from untreated sepsis or hepatitis B (such as recent hepatitis B infection with hepatitis B IgM antibodies or hepatitis B surface-antigen-positive donors without hepatitis B core antibodies)), medical disease (such as insulin-dependent diabetes mellitus for more than 5 years), and renal disease (such as in an anuric donor, although these should be considered if they had previous normal function and have suffered acute kidney injury, which may occur with prolonged hypertension or hypotension). There have been discussions regarding the use of marginal donors for children who have been awaiting renal transplantation without the availability of a living donor and are accruing risks from dialysis treatment.

Peritransplantation issues

There needs to be close collaboration between the pediatric nephrologist, transplant surgeon, anesthetist, and intensivist for all patients, but specifically for smaller patients, in meeting blood pressure aims and fluid management. Such recipients will require very aggressive fluid-loading prior to reperfusion of the kidney, in order to avoid an almost inevitable hypoperfusion and, in the worst case, thrombosis; our experience suggests that only anesthetists experienced in renal transplantation are able to manage this safely. The renal artery and vein are anastomosed to the aorta and inferior vena cava (IVC), respectively, for the smallest patients (10–15 kg), who often have midline incisions with a transperitoneal approach, rather than the conventional retroperitoneal approach to the iliac vessels via the iliac fossa. Closure of the abdomen when implanting an adult kidney into a small infant may be difficult but is usually possible; occasionally a right-sided nephrectomy is necessary at the same time, but invariably such recipients require ventilation and management in a pediatric intensive-care unit overnight. Most transplant surgeons would anastomose the ureter to the bladder with a formal antireflux procedure and leave a transplant ureteric stent temporarily through the vesico-ureteric junction. However, some children with hostile bladders may require a ureterostomy or ureteric implantation into an augmented bladder or ileal conduit [3].

Due to the high clinical nursing and medical input required in the early postoperative period, many units arrange for pediatric intensive-care admission for all patients, although this is only done in our unit for ventilated recipients (usually smaller children who are electively ventilated, as noted earlier). Meticulous attention is required for general fluid and electrolyte balance, due to the large volumes of urine that can be passed depending on the native urine output and the quality of the transplanted organ. Serum electrolytes should be assessed at 2–4-hourly intervals in order to avoid the development of potentially fatal complications, such as severe hyponatremia.

There is no standard immunosuppressive regimen for children and adolescents undergoing renal transplantation but all pediatric renal-transplantation units will have their own protocols or be involved in immunosuppressive drug trials (aiming for children to be entered into multicenter international randomized controlled trials). Due to the different etiology of ESRF in children, as well as their comorbidities, surgical complexities, the metabolism of immunosuppression, and the complications of immunosuppressive therapies in a developing immune system, it is inadvisable to extrapolate results from adult randomized controlled data to pediatric programs. Therefore, as in adult practice, individual protocols vary, but most pediatric renal-transplant recipients currently receive triple therapy, with tacrolimus, an antiproliferative agent (azathioprine or mycophenolate mofetil), and prednisolone (although there are corticosteroid-sparing and weaning protocols), with or without an induction agent—usually an anti-CD25 monoclonal antibody, such as basiliximab—as an interleukin-2 receptor antagonist. Induction therapies are usually given to children on corticosteroid avoidance [19,20] or withdrawal [21] protocols or to reduce calcineurin nephrotoxicity exposure, or else they can be given to those with increased immunological risk (such as patients with donor-specific antibodies). Interestingly, there was no additional benefit to the addition of basiliximab to a protocol of corticosteroids, azathioprine, and tacrolimus in a randomized controlled trial in pediatric renal-transplant recipients [22,23]. There are good outcomes, including improved renal function [24] and growth, in corticosteroid-free and withdrawal protocols [25,26]. Pediatric transplantation physicians aim to balance the risks of acute rejection (due to underimmunosuppression) and infection (with the risk of development of EBV-related PTLD due to over-immunosuppression), so regular monitoring for EBV viremia is required for pediatric patients [27]. Longer-term issues such as chronic allograft dysfunction and poor growth require optimization of therapy and tailoring of medications with time post-transplantation in view of comorbidites (such as insulin-requiring NODAT) and therapeutic drug monitoring. Exposure to calcineurin inhibitors is minimized or withdrawn where there is evidence of chronic allograft dysfunction with interstitial fibrosis and/or tubular atrophy on percutaneous renal-transplant biopsy, at which point mycophenolate mofetil therapy can be introduced with monitoring of donor-specific antibodies to ensure that humorally-mediated rejection does not occur [28].

There may be medical or surgical complications attached to transplantation, such as bacterial (including wound and urinary-tract), viral, fungal, protozoal, and other opportunistic infections, and many units still employ co-trimoxazole prophylaxis against *Pneumocystis carinii* for at least 6 months post-transplantation [29]. There may be postoperative ileus, where enteral feeding can be delayed after intraperitoneal surgery. The risk of renal arterial and venous thrombosis is greatest in the first few days post-transplantation and in smaller children, in whom aspirin therapy is usually advocated; this may be augmented with low-molecular-weight heparin if prothrombotic tendencies are identified [30]. Renal-allograft thrombosis may be caused by severe acute rejection, procoagulant state, and/or reduced blood flow due to surgical technique or decreased circulating blood volume. Children usually present with renal allograft dysfunction (including increased plasma creatinine associated with sudden reduction of urine output), macroscopic hematuria (if venous thrombosis), renal-allograft swelling (with resultant pain or tenderness), and thrombocytopenia. There may be no flow on radiological investigations, including Doppler renal-transplant ultrasound (which is carried out early post-transplantation) and nuclear medicine imaging with ^{99m}technetium-labelled diethylene triamine pentaacetic acid (DTPA) or mercaptoacetyltriglycine (MAG3). Due to the fact that the transplanted kidney does not have collaterals to maintain its blood supply, treatment is surgical, with graft nephrectomy. Other vascular complications may include vascular disease from donors, vascular steal syndrome—where patients have claudication of the affected limb due to narrowing of the iliac vessels—and transplant renal-artery stenosis, which may result from damage to the donor or recipient vessel by clamp injury, kinking of the renal artery, or vessel injury from the perfusion catheter. Initial investigation is by Doppler transplant renal ultrasound followed by angiography (or nuclear medicine imaging with DTPA scans in some centers). Digital subtraction angiography is preferred over computerized tomography (CT) or magnetic resonance angiography (MRA) where there is a high index of suspicion, as this can be an investigational and therapeutic interventional procedure.

There may be hemorrhage (from use of aspirin and/or heparin to prevent renal-allograft thrombosis) or lymphocoeles, due to lymphatic leakage from vessels dissected around the blood vessels at the time of transplantation, although this appears to be more common with the use of sirolimus and everolimus. Lymphocoeles may be asymptomatic and diagnosed on ultrasound, but patients can present with swollen lower limbs due to obstruction of venous return or ureteric obstruction of transplant drainage. Aspiration, ablation using tetracycline, and/or internal drainage by "marsupialization" (which can be performed laparoscopically) might also be considered. There may be urinary leaks at the vesico-ureteric junction due to compromised ureteric blood flow or occasionally a ruptured calyx, when patients may present with abdominal pain and renal allograft dysfunction (due to absorption or falling plasma creatinine with relative oliguria), and investigations can delineate abdominal collections on ultrasound, bladder leaks on cystogram or DTPA, and aspirated fluid for biochemical analysis. Renal-transplant recipients should have bladder catheterization in order to allow the leak to heal, although surgery may be required in a minority of cases. Obstruction of the transplant ureter may occur initially post-transplantation due to lymphocoele or clots, or latterly due to vesico-ureteric-junction obstruction, nephrolithiasis, or ureteric stenosis, which may be caused by BK polyomaviral infection or ischemic injury, as the ureter has a tenuous blood supply. Transplant ureteric obstruction is diagnosed by transplant renal ultrasound with nuclear medicine imaging using DTPA or MAG3, with furosemide or antegrade studies if necessary, and is treated by surgical repair or endoscopically by dilatation if the short narrowed segment is under 2 cm.

Renal-transplant recipients are usually discharged from hospital when lines are removed and they no longer require nursing care in order to administer their own fluid, medication, and catheterization (if indicated) requirements. This can be 1 week after a living related renal transplantation, but may be delayed in cases of primary nonfunction or delayed graft function requiring dialysis therapy in a deceased-donor renal transplantation (although usually, with primary function, patients can be discharged at around 10 days).

Post-transplantation care

Post-transplantation management involves monitoring clinical progress and renal-allograft function and reducing the incidence of complications such as acute rejection and infections in pediatric renal-transplant recipients. The frequency of outpatient visits will be decided locally as part of a protocol of shared care from the specialized pediatric transplantation and local units, but will be individualized according to the renal-allograft function, complications encountered in the initial post-transplant period, and the development of modifiable risk factors (such as CKD parameters with renal-allograft dysfunction (measurement of plasma creatinine and estimation and formal measurement of glomerular filtration rate $(ml/minute/1.73\,m^2)$), hypertension, proteinuria, hyperlipidemia, hyperglycemia, secondary hyperparathyroidism, and donor-specific antibodies) specific to each renal-transplant recipient [31].

The initial follow-up will be very frequent: up to several times per week in the first month post-transplantation. This will be reduced in patients without chronic allograft dysfunction a few years post-renal transplantation, although usually not to more than quarterly. However, patients should have direct access to the pediatric renal-transplantation team in case of emergencies with intercurrent infections or with symptoms or signs of acute rejection.

The aim of intensive follow-up is to improve the long-term patient and renal-allograft outcomes in order to increase the half-life of transplanted kidneys to 20 years [32]. Early identification and successful management of recurrence of primary disease will increase renal-allograft survival [33]. Ongoing monitoring of renal-allograft function will help identify signs of chronic allograft dysfunction, which can lead to intervention and improved outcome [34]. The medical and psychosocial needs of patients and their families can be identified early with the involvement of the multidisciplinary team, which can lead to ongoing education with respect to adherence to fluids, medications, catheterization, outpatient appointments, and investigations to improve long-term outcomes and increase quality of life [35]. This is particularly important in adolescents as they go through the transition process and eventual transfer to adult renal-transplantation centers [36,37]. There should be ongoing programs to educate patients regarding reducing the risk of infection (with routine annual influenza (including H1N1) vaccination and sexual-health education), obesity (healthy living advice), smoking, alcohol, and recreational drug use. There should be active screening surveillance to highlight the importance of applying high-protection-factor sunscreens and examine for a risk of dermatological and other malignancies.

Other aspects of renal transplantation follow-up include improvement of cardiovascular health and ongoing research looking at prospective complications, including cardiac dysfunction [38]. Cardiovascular risk factors may be modifiable through investigations focused on carotid intima media thickness [39], pulse-wave velocity [40], arterial stiffness [41], and left-ventricular mass [42].

Prospective monitoring of pediatric renal-transplant recipients can help early identification of premalignant conditions and malignancy (such as routine EBV PCR DNA testing for EBV viremia and the development of EBV-driven PTLD) [43].

The future of pediatric transplantation

Many pediatric renal-transplantation centers are expanding due to the increased number of children presenting with ESRF and patients who were initially transplanted as infants requiring retransplantation for failing renal transplants with chronic allograft dysfunction, which may be associated with the presence of donor-specific antibodies and C4d-positive immunohistochemistry staining on percutaneous renal-transplant biopsy.

International researchers are investigating the use of biomarkers for acute rejection, as by the time renal-allograft dysfunction with increased plasma creatinine has been identified, there may already be irreversible damage. Some authors are advocating protocol renal-transplant biopsies (although at present there is no consensus on treatment of subclinical rejection) and gene arrays for diagnosing rejection [44,45], with the utilization of rituximab as a chimeric anti-CD20 monoclonal antibody for treating antibody-mediated acute rejection episodes [46].

Another aspect to pediatric renal transplantation is the prophylaxis, active surveillance, and early identification and treatment of viral infections (such as cytomegalovirus (CMV) and EBV). Pediatric renal-transplant recipients are monitored for the presence of EBV viremia in order to reduce immunosuppression and thus the risk of developing PTLD. Initial studies have been unable to identify a useful EBV vaccine [47], although further studies are currently underway with other EBV and CMV vaccinations.

Some children have already received two or three renal transplants, and transplantion of the "untransplantable" is being considered following the successful treatment of the recurrence of primary disease post-transplantation (such as atypical hemolytic uremic syndrome with eculizumab, and focal and segmental glomerulosclerosis with rituximab), following ABO-incompatible renal transplantation, and following desensitization programs for HLA-incompatible transplants and those with high titers of donor-specific antibodies.

These increasing treatments aim to improve the long-term outcomes of children with ESRF by providing them with successful initial and subsequent renal transplants in order to ensure that they have an increased quality and quantity of life.

References

1 Marks SD. How have the past 5 years of research changed clinical practice in paediatric nephrology? *Arch Dis Child* 2007;92(4):357–361.

2 Lewis MA, Shaw J, Sinha M, Adalat S, Hussain F, Inward C. Demography of the UK paediatric renal replacement therapy population. In: Ansell D, Feehally J, Fogarty D, Tomson C, Williams AJ, Warwick G (eds). *The Renal Association and UK Renal Registry—The Eleventh Annual Report*. 2009. pp. 257–267.

3 Riley P, Marks SD, Desai DY, Mushtaq I, Koffman G, Mamode N. Challenges facing renal transplantation in pediatric patients with lower urinary tract dysfunction. *Transplantation* 2010;89(11):1299–1307.

4 Weber S, Moriniere V, Knuppel T, Charbit M, Dusek J, Ghiggeri GM, *et al.* Prevalence of mutations in renal developmental genes in children with renal hypodysplasia: results of the ESCAPE study. *J Am Soc Nephrol*; 17(10): 2864–2870.

5 O'Toole JF, Otto EA, Hoefele J, Helou J, Hildebrandt F. Mutational analysis in 119 families with nephronophthisis. *Pediatr Nephrol* 2007;22(3):366–370.

6 Ajzensztejn MJ, Sebire NJ, Trompeter RS, Marks SD. Primary hyperoxaluria type 1. *Arch Dis Child* 2007;92(3):197.

7 Benden C, Kansra S, Ridout DA, Shaw NL, Aurora P, Elliott MJ, *et al.* Chronic kidney disease in children following lung and heart-lung transplantation. *Pediatr Transplant* 2009;13(1):104–110.

8 Papalois VE, Moss A, Gillingham KJ, Sutherland DE, Matas AJ, Humar A. Pre-emptive transplants for patients with renal failure: an argument against waiting until dialysis. *Transplantation* 2000;70(4):625–631.

9 Meister MG, Olsen OE, de BR, McHugh K, Marks SD. What is the value of magnetic resonance venography in children before renal transplantation? *Pediatr Nephrol* 2008;23(7):1157–1162.

10 Genberg H, Kumlien G, Wennberg L, Berg U, Tyden G. ABO-incompatible kidney transplantation using antigen-specific immunoadsorption and rituximab: a 3-year follow-up. *Transplantation* 2008;85(12):1745–1754.

11 Shishido S, Asanuma H, Tajima E, Hoshinaga K, Ogawa O, Hasegawa A, *et al.* ABO-incompatible living-donor kidney transplantation in children. *Transplantation* 2001;72(6):1037–1042.

12 Shishido S, Hasegawa A. Current status of ABO-incompatible kidney transplantation in children. *Pediatr Transplant* 2005;9(2):148–154.

13 Mamode N, Marks SD. *Maximising living donation with paediatric blood-group-incompatible renal transplantation*. Pediatr Nephrol 2012; in press.

14 Kramer A, Stel VS, Tizard J, Verrina E, Ronnholm K, Palsson R, *et al.* Characteristics and survival of young adults who started renal replacement therapy during childhood. *Nephrol Dial Transplant* 2009;24(3):926–933.

15 Rabbat CG, Thorpe KE, Russell JD, Churchill DN. Comparison of mortality risk for dialysis patients and cadaveric first renal transplant recipients in Ontario, Canada. *J Am Soc Nephrol* 2000;11(5):917–922.

16 Wong CS, Hingorani S, Gillen DL, Sherrard DJ, Watkins SL, Brandt JR, *et al.* Hypoalbuminemia and risk of death in pediatric patients with end-stage renal disease. *Kidney Int* 2002;61(2):630–637.

17 Farid SG, Goldsmith PJ, Fisher J, Feather S, Finlay E, Attia M, *et al.* Successful outcome of paediatric en bloc kidney transplantation from the youngest donation-after-cardiac-death donor in the United Kingdom. *Transpl Int* 2009;22(7):761–762.

18 Jones HE, Drage M, Marks SD. Successful en bloc donation after circulatory death renal transplant into paediatric recipients. *Pediatr Nephrol* 2012;27(9):1817–1818.

19 Li L, Chang A, Naesens M, Kambham N, Waskerwitz J, Martin J, *et al.* Steroid-free immunosuppression since 1999: 129 pediatric renal transplants with sustained graft and patient benefits. *Am J Transplant* 2009;9(6):1362–1372.

20 Sutherland S, Li L, Concepcion W, Salvatierra O, Sarwal MM. Steroid-free immunosuppression in pediatric renal transplantation: rationale for and [corrected] outcomes following conversion to steroid based therapy. *Transplantation* 2009;87(11):1744–1748.

21 Hocker B, Weber LT, Feneberg R, Drube J, John U, Fehrenbach H, *et al.* Prospective, randomized trial on late steroid withdrawal in pediatric renal transplant recipients under cyclosporine microemulsion and mycophenolate mofetil. *Transplantation* 2009;87(6):934–941.

22 Grenda R, Watson A, Vondrak K, Webb NJ, Beattie J, Fitzpatrick M, *et al.* A prospective, randomized, multicenter trial of tacrolimus-based therapy with or without basiliximab in pediatric renal transplantation. *Am J Transplant* 2006;6(7):1666–1672.

23 Webb NJ, Prokurat S, Vondrak K, Watson AR, Hughes DA, Marks SD, *et al.* Multicentre prospective randomised trial of tacrolimus, azathioprine and prednisolone with or without basiliximab: two-year follow-up data. *Pediatr Nephrol* 2009;24(1):177–182.

24 Li L, Weintraub L, Concepcion W, Martin JP, Miller K, Salvatierra O, *et al.* Potential influence of tacrolimus and steroid avoidance on early graft function in pediatric renal transplantation. *Pediatr Transplant* 2008;12(6):701–707.

25 Grenda R. Effects of steroid avoidance and novel protocols on growth in paediatric renal transplant patients. *Pediatr Nephrol* 2010;25(4):747–752.

26 Grenda R, Watson A, Trompeter R, Tonshoff B, Jaray J, Fitzpatrick M *et al.* A randomized trial to assess the impact of early steroid withdrawal on growth in pediatric renal transplantation: the TWIST study. *Am J Transplant* 2010; 10(4):828–836.

27 Krischock L, Marks SD. Induction therapy: why, when, and which agent? *Pediatr Transplant* 2010;14(3):298–313.

28 Krischock L, Gullett A, Bockenhauer D, Rees L, Trompeter RS, Marks SD. Calcineurin-inhibitor free immunosuppression with mycophenolate mofetil and corticosteroids in paediatric renal transplantation improves renal allograft function without increasing acute rejection. *Pediatr Transplant* 2009; 13(4):475–481.

29 Mencarelli F, Marks SD. Non-viral infections in children after transplantation. *Pediatr Nephrol* 2012;27(9):1465–1476.

30 Nagra A, Trompeter RS, Fernando ON, Koffman G, Taylor JD, Lord R, *et al.* The effect of heparin on graft thrombosis in pediatric renal allografts. *Pediatr Nephrol* 2004;19(5):531–535.

31 Sinha R, Saad A, Marks SD. Prevalence and complications of chronic kidney disease in paediatric renal transplantation: a K/DOQI perspective. *Nephrol Dial Transplant* 2010;25(4):1313–1320.

32 Rees L, Shroff R, Hutchinson C, Fernando ON, Trompeter RS. Long-term outcome of paediatric renal transplantation: follow-up of 300 children from 1973 to 2000. *Nephron Clin Pract* 2007;105(2):c68–c76.

33 Cochat P, Fargue S, Mestrallet G, Jungraithmayr T, Koch-Nogueira P, Ranchin B, *et al*. Disease recurrence in paediatric renal transplantation. *Pediatr Nephrol* 2009;24(11):2097–2108.

34 Fletcher JT, Nankivell BJ, Alexander SI. Chronic allograft nephropathy. *Pediatr Nephrol* 2009;24(8):1465–1471.

35 Riano-Galan I, Malaga S, Rajmil L, Ariceta G, Navarro M, Loris C, *et al*. Quality of life of adolescents with end-stage renal disease and kidney transplant. *Pediatr Nephrol* 2009;24(8):1561–1568.

36 Bell L. Adolescents with renal disease in an adult world: meeting the challenge of transition of care. *Nephrol Dial Transplant* 2007;22(4):988–991.

37 Harden PN, Walsh G, Bandler N, Bradley S, Lonsdale D, Taylor J, Marks SD. Bridging the gap: an integrated paediatric to adult clinical service for young adults with kidney failure. *BMJ* 2012;344:e3718.

38 Kim GB, Kwon BS, Kang HG, Ha JW, Ha IS, Noh CI, *et al*. Cardiac dysfunction after renal transplantation; incomplete resolution in pediatric population. *Transplantation* 2009;87(11):1737–1743.

39 Delucchi A, Dinamarca H, Gainza H, Whitttle C, Torrealba I, Iniguez G. Carotid intima-media thickness as a cardiovascular risk marker in pediatric end-stage renal disease patients on dialysis and in renal transplantation. *Transplant Proc* 2008;40(9):3244–3246.

40 Cseprekal O, Kis E, Schaffer P, Othmane TH, Fekete BC, Vannay A, *et al*. Pulse wave velocity in children following renal transplantation. *Nephrol Dial Transplant* 2009;24(1):309–315.

41 Briese S, Claus M, Querfeld U. Arterial stiffness in children after renal transplantation. *Pediatr Nephrol* 2008;23(12):2241–2245.

42 Becker-Cohen R, Nir A, Ben-Shalom E, Rinat C, Feinstein S, Farber B, *et al*. Improved left ventricular mass index in children after renal transplantation. *Pediatr Nephrol* 2008;23(9):1545–1550.

43 Koukourgianni F, Harambat J, Ranchin B, Euvrard S, Bouvier R, Liutkus A, *et al*. Malignancy incidence after renal transplantation in children: a 20-year single-centre experience. *Nephrol Dial Transplant* 2010;25(2):611–616.

44 Khatri P, Sarwal MM. Using gene arrays in diagnosis of rejection. *Curr Opin Organ Transplant* 2009;14(1):34–39.

45 Zarkhin V, Sarwal MM. Microarrays: monitoring for transplant tolerance and mechanistic insights. *Clin Lab Med* 2008;28(3):385–410, vi.

46 Zarkhin V, Li L, Kambham N, Sigdel T, Salvatierra O, Sarwal MM. A randomized, prospective trial of rituximab for acute rejection in pediatric renal transplantation. *Am J Transplant* 2008;8(12):2607–2617.

47 Rees L, Tizard EJ, Morgan AJ, Cubitt WD, Finerty S, Oyewole-Eletu TA, *et al*. A phase I trial of epstein-barr virus gp350 vaccine for children with chronic kidney disease awaiting transplantation. *Transplantation* 2009;88(8):1025–1029.

10 Immunosuppressive Pharmacotherapy

Steven Gabardi[1] and Anil Chandraker[2]

[1] Renal Division/Departments of Transplant Surgery and Pharmacy Services, Brigham and Women's Hospital; and Department of Medicine, Harvard Medical School, USA
[2] Renal Division, Brigham and Women's Hospital, Harvard Medical School, USA

Introduction

Optimal pharmacological management of renal transplant recipients (RTRs) is imperative when attempting to achieve long-term patient and allograft survival. Short-term outcomes of transplantation have improved considerably over the past 3 decades, due in large part to a more robust understanding of immunology and improvements in surgical techniques, organ procurement, immunosuppression, and post-transplant care [1]. Despite the improvements in short-term survival, late graft loss and complications of long-term immunosuppression remain a concern.

In transplantation, clinical immunosuppression is an empirical practice whose primary goal is to prevent acute rejection while limiting harm to the patient or allograft. Unfortunately, this practice is fraught with imprecision due to the lack of a satisfactory in vivo technique for determining the degree of immunosuppression in patients. Inadequate immunosuppression can result in allograft rejection, whereas overimmunosuppression can lead to significant adverse events, including infection and malignancy. The adverse-event profiles of the individual immunosuppressants necessitate intense post-transplant patient monitoring. Although local protocols and national/international guidelines have been developed to help streamline immunosuppressive strategies, each patient must be managed individually, with constant, careful adjustments of their immunosuppressive and nonimmunosuppressive medications.

Most immunosuppressive protocols are based on the premise that following the transplant, the immune response is at its most vigorous and will require maximal suppression. Over time, host–graft adaptation occurs and less immunosuppression is needed. However, determining the appropriate level of immunosuppression in different patients over time remains difficult. Consequently, most immunosuppressive protocols begin with induction therapy and/or high doses of maintenance immunosuppression in the critical, early post-transplantation period. The doses of maintenance

Abdominal Organ Transplantation: State of the Art, First Edition.
Edited by Nizam Mamode and Raja Kandaswamy.

immunosuppression can be steadily reduced over time to a level that the practitioner feels is appropriate for the given patient. In order for this to best be accomplished, it is imperative that clinicians be aware of the specific advantages and disadvantages of the available immunosuppressants, as well as the potential for drug misadventure commonly seen with these agents. This chapter will review the currently available immunosuppressive agents and potential future immunosuppressants, focusing on their pharmacology, dosing, adverse-event profile, drug–drug interaction (DDI), and clinical efficacy.

Immunosuppressive therapies

Most immunosuppressive regimens are built utilizing multiple agents, all working on different immunological targets. The primary reason for a multidrug regimen is to allow for pharmacological activity at several key steps in the T-cell activation/replication process; however, this type of regimen employs lower doses of each individual agent, resulting in less drug-related toxicity.

The three stages of clinical immunosuppression are induction therapy, maintenance therapy, and management of acute rejection. The immunosuppressive therapies used for each of these stages will be discussed in detail in this section. Figure 10.1 depicts the location of action of the current immunosuppressive therapies and immunosuppressants in clinical trials.

Induction therapy

Induction therapy provides a high level of immunosuppression in the early post-transplant period, when the risk of acute rejection is highest [2]. This

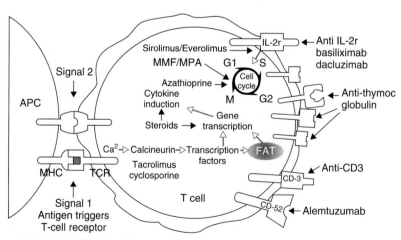

Figure 10.1 Locations of action of the current immunosuppressive therapies and immunosuppressants. (Reproduced by permission from John Wiley & Sons Ltd: from [3] Larsen CP, Knechtle SJ, Adams A, Pearson T, and Kirk AD. A Therapeutic Strategy for Long-term Maintenance Immunosuppression. *American Journal of Transplantation* 2006;6(5):876–883)

Table 10.1 Induction agents used in renal transplant [1,9,28].

Generic name (brand name)	Depleting/ nondepleting	Dosing[a]	Common adverse events
Basiliximab	Nondepleting	20 mg IV × 2 doses	None reported compared to placebo
Antithymocyte globulin equine (ATGe)	Depleting	15 mg/kg/day IV × 3–14 days	Flu-like symptoms, gastrointestinal (GI) distress, rash, back pain, myelosuppression
Antithymocyte globulin rabbit (ATGr)	Depleting	1.5 mg/kg/day IV × 3–14 days	Flu-like symptoms, GI distress, rash, generalized pain, myelosuppression
Alemtuzumab	Depleting	30 mg IV × 1–2 doses	Flu-like symptoms, GI distress, dizziness, myelosuppression

[a]If the common dose is weight-based then a dose was calculated based on a 70 kg patient.
IV, intravenous

stage of immunosuppression is not obligatory; however, given the impact of acute rejection on long-term allograft function, induction therapy is often considered essential to optimum outcome. This is especially true in patients at high immunological risk for rejection. Induction-therapy agents (Table 10.1) are classified as either monoclonal or polyclonal antibodies. Even so, based on their mechanisms of action, these agents may be more clearly delineated by categorizing them as either depleting (OKT3, antithymocyte globulins (ATGs), alemtuzumab) or nondepleting (basiliximab, daclizumab) proteins [2].

The primary reason for using induction therapy is that these agents are highly immunosuppressive, which allows for a significant reduction in acute rejections rates and improved 1-year graft survival [2,4]. Additionally, these agents are often considered essential for use in patients at high risk for poor short-term outcomes, such as those with preformed antibodies, a history of previous organ transplants, multiple human leukocyte antigen (HLA) mismatches, or who have received organ transplants with prolonged cold-ischemic time or from expanded-criteria donors and donors after cardiac death. Induction therapy can also play an important role in preventing early-onset calcineurin inhibitor (CNI)-induced nephrotoxicity [2,4]. With the use of induction therapy, CNI initiation can often be delayed until the graft regains some function [5].

The short-term improvements in outcomes gained from the use of induction therapies are undeniable, and are discussed in this section, yet studies detailing the impact of induction therapy on long-term allograft function or survival are needed. Practitioners should realize that, when using these highly immunosuppressive agents—particularly the depleting proteins (also known as the antilymphocyte antibodies (ALAs))—host defenses are profoundly impaired, predisposing patients to opportunistic infections and/or malignancies.

Declining worldwide use and manufacturing expenses of both OKT3 and daclizumab have led the makers of these agents to discontinue their production [6]. This review will discuss only those induction agents that remain available.

Nondepleting protein (basiliximab)
Pharmacology
Basiliximab is a chimeric monoclonal antibody that binds with high affinity to and antagonizes the alpha subunit of the interleukin-2 (IL-2) receptor (i.e. CD25) [7,8]. This agent inhibits IL-2-mediated activation of lymphocytes, which is a necessary step in clonal expansion of T-cells [8,9].

Dosing
In adults and children ≥35 kg, intravenous (IV) basiliximab is given at doses of 20 mg 2 hours prior to transplant and again on postoperative day 4 [7,8]. In patients <35 kg, 10 mg doses should be used at the same dosing interval. This dosing strategy saturates CD25 for up to 8 weeks. No dose adjustments are necessary in renal or hepatic dysfunction [7,8].

Adverse events
The incidence of all adverse reactions with basiliximab was similar to placebo in clinical trials [8–10]. On rare occasions (<1% of patients), severe acute hypersensitivity reactions have been reported after both initial exposure and reexposure to this medication. The absence of any increased risk of cytomegalovirus (CMV) infection or malignancy is noteworthy [8–10]. In comparison to induction therapy with ATG, 16 recipients would need therapy with an IL-2-receptor antagonist in order to prevent one case of CMV, and 58 patients would need an IL-2-receptor antagonist to prevent one patient from having malignancy [11].

Depleting proteins (ATGs)
Pharmacology
Polyclonal antibodies directed against human lymphoid tissue are prepared by immunizing animals with human thymocytes [4,7,12,13]. Currently, there are two ATG preparations available in the USA. Antithymocyte globulin equine (eATG) is a purified, concentrated, and sterilized antibody preparation obtained from the hyperimmune serum of horses. This preparation depletes the number of circulating, thymus-dependent lymphocytes through multiple mechanisms. eATG contains antibodies against many T-cell surface markers and promotes T-cell depletion through opsonization with complement-mediated lysis and clearance into the reticuloendothelial system. Immune reconstitution after depletion with eATG takes several months. Overall, the number of lymphocytes in the peripheral circulation, the thymus, and the spleen is reduced [5,7,12,13].

Antithymocyte globulin rabbit (rATG) is also a cytolytic polyclonal antibody preparation [4,7,13]. It is a purified and pasteurized preparation of gamma immunoglobulin derived by immunizing rabbits with human thymocytes. Possible mechanisms by which rATG induces immunosuppression in vivo include T-cell clearance from the circulation and modulation of T-cell activation, homing, and cytotoxic activities. In vitro, rATG mediates T-cell suppressive effects via inhibition of proliferative responses to several mitogens. rATG is thought to induce T-cell depletion and modulation by a variety of methods, including Fc receptor-mediated complement-dependent lysis, opsonization and phagocytosis by macrophages, and immunomodulation leading to long-term depletion via apoptosis and antibody-dependent cell-mediated cytotoxicity. Cell recovery may take several months following rATG administration [4,7,13]. It has been shown that T-cell recovery following rATG-induced depletion is associated with an expansion of suppressor T-cells, potentially inducing long-term immunomodulation [14].

Dosing

The approved induction-therapy dosing strategy for eATG is 10–30 mg/kg/day IV for 7–14 days [5,7,12,13]. The initial dose should be administered shortly before or after transplantation. In many instances, this prolonged course is associated with a difficult outpatient administration and high cost. A shorter course of therapy (15 mg/kg/day for 7–10 days) is often used to counter these issues. rATG is not approved for induction therapy but is routinely used for this purpose. When used in this capacity, rATG has been dosed at 1–4 mg/kg/day for 3–10 days after transplantation. The most common dosing regimen with this agent is four doses of 1.5 mg/kg/day, resulting in a total dosage of 6 mg/kg over the course of therapy [4,7,13]. There is a benefit in giving the initial dose intraoperatively prior to the anastamosis of the renal artery in order to reduce organ reperfusion injury [15].

Adverse events

Cytokine release-related adverse events, such as fever, chills, headache, back pain, nausea, diarrhea, dizziness, malaise, and myelosuppression, are common with both ATG preparations [7]. ATG-treated patients experience significantly more fever, cytokine-release syndrome, infusion-related reactions, and leukopenia compared to those patients receiving an IL-2-receptor antagonist [11]. Premedication with an antihistamine and acetaminophen is recommended to lower the incidence of fever and chills during the infusion. Anaphylactic reactions have occurred with the administration of eATG and the manufacturer strongly recommends the administration of a skin test prior to the first dose of eATG to assess the potential for an allergic reaction. The patient and injection site should be examined every 15–20 minutes for 1 hour after the administration of the test dose. Unfortunately, a negative skin test does not completely rule out the potential for an allergic reaction. The strong recommendation of the skin test makes the use of eATG more difficult than other antibody preparations [5,7,12]. A test dose is not recommended when using rATG.

There is a theoretical concern about retreatment with ATG for management of steroid-resistant acute rejection in a patient who received ATG for induction therapy, due to the potential for increased adverse events and allergic reaction. Although this has never been formally analyzed in a prospective, randomized manner, two retrospective case series suggest that readministration of rATG can be safely carried out in RTRs [16,17].

Comparative efficacy (eATG versus rATG)

Brennan *et al.* conducted the sentinel study of eATG versus rATG, in which 72 RTRs were randomized to receive rATG 1.5 mg/kg (n = 48) or eATG 15 mg/kg (n = 24) daily for up to 6 days [18]. All patients were maintained on either cyclosporine (CsA), azathioprine (AZA), and prednisone or CsA, mycophenolate mofetil (MMF), and prednisone. At 12 months, patient survival and renal function were similar between the two groups. However, graft survival was higher with rATG (98%) compared to eATG (83%) (p = 0.020) and acute rejection occurred more frequently with eATG (25%) compared to rATG (4.2% (p = 0.014) at 1 year. In terms of adverse events, leukopenia occurred more commonly with rATG (56.3%) than with eATG (4.2%) (p < 0.0001). Despite this, 6-month CMV disease rates were lower in patients treated with rATG (10%) compared to eATG (33%) (p = 0.025). Post-transplant lymphoproliferative disease (PTLD) did not occur in either group [18].

A 10-year follow-up of these patients revealed that event-free survival (48 versus 29%; p = 0.011) and the incidence of acute rejection (11 versus 42%; p = 0.004) were superior with rATG [19]. Mean serum creatinine levels were higher (1.7 ± 0.5 versus 1.2 ± 0.3 mg/dl; p = 0.003) in the eATG group. There were 0.53 quality-adjusted life years gained from rATG induction [19].

Comparative efficacy (basiliximab versus rATG)

Many have theorized that when using depleting proteins, one has to endure a higher incidence of adverse events in order to attain improved efficacy versus a nondepleting protein. Several studies have attempted to prove this by evaluating the differences between basiliximab and rATG; the most referenced one was carried out by Brennan *et al.* [20]. Per protocol, event-free survival was defined as freedom from a composite endpoint (biopsy-proven acute rejection (BPAR), delayed graft function (DGF), graft loss, and death). Patients were randomized to receive either rATG (1.5 mg/kg/day from day 0 to day 4; n = 141) or basiliximab (20 mg/day on days 0 and 4; n = 137). Maintenance immunosuppression with CsA-modified, MMF, and corticosteroids was given to all patients. At 12 months, the composite endpoint was similar in both groups (rATG = 50.4%, basiliximab = 56.2%; p = 0.34). However, the incidence of BPAR was lower with rATG (15.6%) versus basiliximab (25.5%) (p = 0.02). Myelosuppression occurred more often in the rATG-treated patients. There were more infectious complications seen with rATG compared to basiliximab (85.8 versus 75.2%; p = 0.03). Despite this, CMV infections were significantly more frequent in the basiliximab group (17.5 versus 7.8%; p = 0.02). Five patients in the rATG group and one patient in the basiliximab group developed malignancy [20].

In a recent meta-analysis, when the IL-2-receptor antibodies were ana-lyzed against the ATG preparations it was found that there was no difference in graft loss [11]. Induction with ATG therapy lowered the rates of BPAR at 1 year (eight studies: RR 1.30, 95% CI 1.01–1.67), but with a 75% increase in malignancy (seven studies: RR 0.25, 95% CI 0.07–0.87) and a 32% increase in CMV disease (13 studies: RR 0.68, 95% CI 0.50–0.93). Adverse events, including myelosuppression and cytokine-release syndrome, occurred more often in patients receiving ATG [11].

Depleting proteins (alemtuzumab)
Pharmacology
Alemtuzumab is a recombinant DNA-derived monoclonal antibody directed against the 21–28 kD cell-surface glycoprotein CD52 [7,21]. CD52 is present on nearly all B- and T-lymphocytes, many macrophages, NK cells, and a subpopulation of granulocytes. This agent causes antibody-dependent cell lysis [22]. Lymphocyte depletion with alemtuzumab is rapid and extensive. Lymphocyte counts may take several months to return to pretransplant levels [21].

Dosing
Alemtuzumab is not approved for use in RTRs. There is no consensus on the appropriate dose of alemtuzumab for induction therapy. Early studies used a dose of 20–30 mg IV or subcutaneous on day 0 and again on either day 1 or day 4 post-transplant [22]. However, current studies are evaluating the use of a single 30 mg dose given on postoperative Day 0, theorizing that this dosing regimen will provide similar efficacy, with improved tolerability, to previous dosing strategies [21].

Adverse events
Some common adverse reactions seen with alemtuzumab include anemia, headache, dysthesias, dizziness, nausea, vomiting, diarrhea, myelosuppression, infusion-related reactions, and infection [7]. The use of premedications (e.g. acetaminophen, antihistamines) is advisable, to reduce the incidence of infusion-related reactions [7,21].

One possible concern with alemtuzumab induction is the potential response associated with immune reconstitution. Although data are unavailable in RTRs, a study in multiple sclerosis showed a profound IL-21-driven autoimmune response following alemtuzumab-induced lymphocyte depletion [23]. Further characterization of the immune system following alemtuzumab use in RTRs is needed in order to understand the long-term impact of the use of this agent as induction therapy.

Comparative efficacy
Data exist on alemtuzumab's efficacy and safety in several observational studies, although only a few randomized controlled trials have been published to date in RTRs. The most cited alemtuzumab analysis was performed by Hanaway et al. [24]. In this prospective analysis, patients were randomized to receive alemtuzumab or either basiliximab or rATG. Patients were stratified according to risk, with 139 high-risk patients receiving alemtuzumab (30 mg × 1 dose; n = 70) or rATG (6 mg/kg total dose; n = 69).

In 335 low-risk individuals, alemtuzumab (30 mg × 1 dose; n = 164) or basiliximab (40 mg total dose; n = 171) was administered. At three years post-transplant, BPAR rates in low-risk patients was lower with alemtuzumab compared to basiliximab (10% vs. 22%; p = 0.003). At the same time period, in high-risk individuals, the rates of BPAR were comparable between alemtuzumab and rATG (18% vs. 15%; p = 0.63). Adverse-event rates were comparable among all four treatment groups [24].

Induction therapy: conclusion

Induction therapy with biological agents increased utilization to 82.8% of kidney transplants in the USA in 2009, continuing a 9-year trend [25]. However, there is no universal consensus on the optimal induction agent. The most recent analysis, in 2009, demonstrated that rATG was the most frequently used induction agent in the USA. Depleting antibody therapy was used in 58% of RTRs, about whom information was available. In contrast, the IL-2-receptor antibodies were used in 21.2% of all RTRs [13,25]. Outside of the USA, the UK National Institute for Health and Clinical Excellence (NICE) has recommended the use of basiliximab for induction therapy; however, NICE provides no review or opinion on the use of the ALA agents [26].

Maintenance therapy

The objective of maintenance immunosuppression is to further aid in preventing acute rejection episodes while optimizing long-term patient and allograft survival [1,27]. Immunosuppressants require careful selection and dosage titration to balance the risks of rejection with those of toxicity. The net state of immunosuppression is strongly correlated with the occurrence of some of the most notorious post-transplant adverse events (e.g. infection, malignancy); therefore, it is vital that the degree of immunosuppression be gradually reduced over time [1,27].

During the early years of transplantation there were few choices for maintenance immunosuppression (e.g. AZA, corticosteroids). In the 1980s, the development of CsA revolutionized organ transplantion by reducing rejection rates substantially and improving 1-year graft survival. The evolution of maintenance immunosuppression in the past 2 decades saw an expansion in therapeutic options which further prevent rejection and improve outcomes. The maintenance immunosuppressive agents, in combination with induction therapy, have made it possible to attain acute rejection rates at or below 10% and increase 1-year graft survival above 90%.

There are five distinct classes of maintenance immunosuppressive agent (Table 10.2): CNIs (CsA and TAC), target-of-rapamycin (ToR) inhibitors (sirolimus and everolimus), antiproliferatives (AZA and the mycophenolic acid (MPA) derivatives) co-stimulation blockade (belatacept), and corticosteroids. In general, maintenance immunosuppression is achieved by combining two or more medications from the different classes in order to maximize efficacy and reduce toxicities. Immunosuppressive regimens vary between transplant centers, but most often include a CNI with an adjuvant agent (e.g. ToR inhibitor, antiproliferative), with or without corticosteroids. Selection of appropriate immunosuppressive agents should

Table 10.2 Maintenance immunosuppressive medications [1,9,28].

Generic name	Common initial dosage	Common adverse effects
CsA	4–5 mg/kg twice a day	Neurotoxicity, gingival hyperplasia, hirsutism, hypertension, hyperlipidemia, glucose intolerance, nephrotoxicity, electrolyte abnormalities
TAC	0.05–0.075 mg/kg twice a day	Neurotoxicity, alopecia, hypertension, hyperlipidemia, glucose intolerance, nephrotoxicity, electrolyte abnormalities
AZA	1.0–2.5 mg/kg once a day	Myelosuppression, gastrointestinal disturbances, pancreatitis
MMF	0.5–1.5 g twice a day	Myelosuppression, gastrointestinal disturbances
EC-MPA	720 mg twice a day	Myelosuppression, gastrointestinal disturbances
Sirolimus	1–10 mg once a day	Hypertriglyceridemia, myelosuppression, mouth sores, hypercholesterolemia, gastrointestinal disturbances, impaired wound-healing, lymphocele, pneumonitis
Everolimus	0.75 mg twice a day	Hypertriglyceridemia, myelosuppression, mouth sores, hypercholesterolemia, gastrointestinal disturbances, impaired wound-healing, lymphocele, pneumonitis
Belatacept	Initial Dosing: 10 mg/kg on post-op days 1 and 4, and post-po weeks 2, 4, 6, 8 and 12. Maintenance Dosing: 5 mg/kg starting at the end of week 16 post-transplant and every four weeks thereafter.	Gastrointestinal disturbances, hyper/hypokalemia, headache, peripheral erdema, anemia, leukopenia, hypotension, arthralgia, insomnia.
Prednisone	Maintenance: 2.5–20.0 mg once a day	Mood disturbances, psychosis, cataracts, hypertension, fluid retention, peptic ulcers, osteoporosis, muscle weakness, impaired wound-healing, glucose intolerance, weight gain, hyperlipidemia

be patient-specific, and transplant practitioners must take into account the immunosuppressive medication's pharmacological properties, adverse event profile, and potential for DDIs, as well as the patient's comorbidities.

CNIs
Pharmacology
The CNIs induce immunosuppression by first complexing with cytoplasmic proteins: CsA with cyclophilin and TAC with FK-binding protein-12 (FKBP-12) [1,7,28]. This complex then binds to and deactivates calcineurin phosphatase, subsequently preventing the dephosphorylation and translocation of nuclear factor of activated T-cells (NFAT). Inhibition of

NFAT's passage through the nuclear membrane reduces the expression of several cytokine genes that promote T-cell activation and expansion, including IL-2, IL-4, interferon-gamma (INF-γ), and tumor necrosis factor-alpha (TNF-α). The end result of inhibiting calcineurin phosphatase is a reduction in cytokine synthesis, with a resultant decline in lymphocyte proliferation [1,7,28].

Pharmaceutics and dosing

CsA is available in two formulations that have very different oral absorption characteristics. The original, oil-based formulation has bile-dependent absorption, resulting in highly variable oral bioavailability. The newer, modified microemulsion formulation has an improved absorption profile that provides a more consistent drug exposure [29]. CsA-modified is the preferred formulation for transplant centers that utilize CsA-based maintenance therapy. The two formulations are not bioequivalent; however, conversion between the two formulations is safe with proper therapeutic drug monitoring (TDM). The labeled initial oral adult dose of CsA following renal transplant is 15 mg/kg/day (range of 8–18 mg/kg/day) administered in two divided doses [1,7,28]. The IV formulation of CsA is used less frequently in renal transplantation due to its high risk of nephrotoxicity. TAC is commercially available in oral and IV formulations. The recommended adult oral dose of TAC following renal transplant is 0.2 mg/kg/day (range of 0.1–0.3 mg/kg/day) administered in two divided doses [1,7,28]. The use of IV TAC carries the risk of anaphylaxis, secondary to its hydrogenated castor-oil component [7]. CNIs should be initiated within 24 hours of transplantation in patients not receiving induction therapy. However, when used in conjunction with induction therapy, dosing may be delayed until some degree of kidney function is seen. The appropriate selection of a starting dose is influenced by the patient's immunological risk, preexisting disease state, and concomitant immunosuppressants. In rare instances, TAC may be given sublingually if gut absorption is questionable, and concern exists regarding the use of IV TAC [30,31]. A once-daily, extended-release TAC formulation has been approved in some European countries and Canada, but has not yet been approved for use in the USA.

Therapeutic drug monitoring

Monitoring whole-blood CsA and TAC levels is imperative, especially early post-transplantation, given the great interpatient and intrapatient variability of these agents [8–10]. Trough levels (C_0) have been the standard monitoring parameter for both CsA and TAC [9,10]. However, for CsA, newer literature has shown that trough concentrations may not have the best correlation with either efficacy or toxicity and suggests that CsA area-under-the-curve (AUC) is best predicted by a 2-hour post-dose (C_2) [9–11]. Since C_2 levels are drawn shortly after the administration, the serum concentrations are much higher when compared to C_0 (800–1500 ng/ml) [9,10]. The long-term benefits of C_2 monitoring remain unclear, yet short-term data suggest that it may provide an initial improvement in renal function and reduce the frequency and severity of CsA-induced hypertension. Manufacturer recommendations for CsA and TAC trough levels range from 50 to 400 ng/ml and from 4 to 20 ng/ml, respectively, depending on the degree of the patient's immunological risk and the time elapsed since the transplant [7]. Many practitioners have argued that the upper limit of trough levels for TAC are too high, as several studies have shown excellent efficacy and safety with levels of less than 12 ng/ml [9]. Target level recommendations are institution- and patient-specific. CNI TDM should not begin until steady state has been reached, which generally occurs 3–4 days after initiation of therapy or dosage change [8–10].

Adverse events

The CNIs have an extensive adverse event profile, with most toxicities being dose-dependent. One of the most infamous effects of both CNIs is their ability to cause nephrotoxicity, as well as other common adverse effects including neurotoxicity, cardiovascular disease, and hyperglycemia [2,4,13]. Rarely, thrombotic thrombocytopenic purpura-hemolytic uremic syndrome can occur while patients are receiving either CNI [32–35]. There are differences between the two agents in terms of adverse-event profiles, which may influence the choice of one agent over the other. For example, post-transplant diabetes, alopecia, and neuropathies are more associated with TAC, while gingival hyperplasia, hirsutism, and hypertension are more commonly associated with CsA. Table 10.3 reviews common CNI adverse events and recommendations for their management.

Comparative efficacy

Several studies have attempted to evaluate the differences between CsA and TAC. A meta-analysis was published in an attempt to differentiate the relative efficacy and safety of the CNIs in RTRs [36]. This report evaluated 30 randomized controlled trials, including more than 4100 patients. This analysis demonstrated that at 6 months post-transplant, TAC was associated with a significantly reduced rate of allograft loss (RR 0.56, 95% CI 0.36–0.86). This benefit was seen for up to 3 years post-transplant, but was diminished in patients in whom higher TAC trough levels were targeted. This advantage over CsA was independent of the formulation of CsA used. TAC was also associated with a reduction in the incidence of BPAR (RR 0.69, 95% CI 0.60–0.79) and steroid-resistant rejection (RR 0.49, 95% CI 0.37–0.64) at 12 months. In terms of safety, TAC was associated with a higher risk of PTDM, neurological effects, and gastrointestinal (GI) disorders, and CsA was associated with more cosmetic-related adverse events and hyperlipidemia [36].

Avoiding CNIs

The fact that CNIs decrease the risk of rejection and improve short-term outcomes in kidney transplantation is undeniable. Despite this, the focus has shifted towards new strategies by which to optimize patient outcomes by preventing CNI-related toxicities. A brief review of some CNI avoidance, minimization, and withdrawal trials is detailed here.

The largest randomized controlled trial to date is the Efficacy Limiting Toxicity Eliminations (ELITE) SYMPHONY trial, which studied the efficacy

Table 10.3 Management of common adverse events associated with the CNIs [1,7,28].

Adverse event	Most likely offending CNI	Monitoring parameters	Therapeutic management options
Alopecia	TAC	• Patient complaints of excessive hair loss	• Reduce TAC dose (if possible) • Hair-growth treatments (e.g. minoxidil, finasteride for males only) • Change from TAC to CsA or sirolimus
CNS toxicities[a]	TAC	• Fine hand tremor • Headache • Mental-status changes	• Reduce TAC dose (if possible) • Change from TAC to CsA or sirolimus
Electrolyte imbalance	Either	• K (usually ↑) • Mg (usually ↓) • PO4 (usually ↓)	• Treat electrolyte imbalance (e.g. Mg replacement) • Reduce CI dose (if possible) • Modify regimen (add or change to non-CI-containing regimen)
GI distress[a]	TAC	• Patient complaints of nausea, vomiting, or diarrhea	• GI distress is often blamed on mycophenolate; this agent may be dose-reduced prior to changing the TAC dose • Reduce TAC dose (if possible) • Change from TAC to CsA or sirolimus
Gingival hyperplasia	CsA	• Patient complaints of excessive gum growth • Recommendations for therapy from the patient's dentist	• Reduce CsA dose (if possible) • Oral surgery (gum resection) • Change from CsA to TAC or sirolimus
Hematologic	Either	• White-blood-cell count • Platelets • Hemoglobin • Hematocrit • Symptoms of anemia	• Reduce CI dose (if possible) • Modify regimen (add or change to non-CI-containing regimen—although hematologic risks are high for all medicines, except steroids)
Hepatotoxicity	Either	• Liver-function tests	• Reduce CI dose (if possible) • Modify regimen (add or change to non-CI-containing regimen)

Table 10.3 (*continued*)

Adverse event	Most likely offending CNI	Monitoring parameters	Therapeutic management options
Hirsutism	CsA	• Patient complaints of excessive hair growth or male-pattern hair growth	• Reduce CsA dose (if possible) • Employ cosmetic hair removal • Change from CsA to TAC or sirolimus
Hyperglycemia[a]	TAC	• Blood glucose (fasting and nonfasting) • HgA1c	• Modify diet • Reduce steroids (if patient is taking them and if possible) • Reduce TAC dose (if possible) • Initiate patient-specific glucose-lowering therapy (insulin or oral therapy) • Change from TAC to CsA or sirolimus
Hyperlipidemia[b]	CsA	• Fasting lipid panel	• Initiate patient-specific cholesterol-lowering therapy • Reduce CsA dose (if possible) • Change from CsA to TAC
Hypertension[b]	CsA	• Blood pressure • Heart rate	• Initiate patient-specific antihypertensive therapy • Reduce CsA dose (if possible) • Change from CsA to TAC or sirolimus
Hyperuricemia	CsA	• Uric acid levels • Patient complaints of a gout flare	• Initiate hyperuricemia treatment (allopurinol, probenecid, colchicines for a gout flare) • Avoid NSAID use, if possible, for symptomatic relief of a gout flare • Reduce CsA dose (if possible) • Change from CsA to TAC or sirolimus
Nephrotoxicity	Either	• Serum creatinine • BUN • Urine output • Biopsy-proven CI-induced nephrotoxicity	• Reduce CI dose (if possible) • Use CCB for HTN control • Modify regimen (add or change to non-CI-containing regimen)

(continued overleaf)

Table 10.3 (*continued*)

Adverse event	Most likely offending CNI	Monitoring parameters	Therapeutic management options
TTP-HUS	Either	• Serum creatinine • Platelet count • Neurological abnormalities • Red-cell fragmentation observed on peripheral blood smear	• Modify regimen (change to non-CI-containing regimen, such as belatacept) • Treat the TTP-HUS (e.g. glucocorticoids, plasma exchange, etc.)

[a]CsA is also associated with CNS toxicities, GI distress, and hyperglycemia, but to a lower extent than TAC.
[b]TAC is also associated with hyperlipidemia and hypertension, but to a lower extent than CsA.
BUN, blood urea nitrogen; CCB, calcium channel blocker; CI, CNI; GI, gastrointestinal; HTN, hypertension; K, potassium; Mg, magnesium; NSAID, nonsteroidal anti-inflammatory drugs; PO4, phosphate; TTP–HUS, thrombotic thrombocytopenic purpura–hemolytic uremic syndrome.

and safety of de novo CNI avoidance in RTRs (n = 1645) [37]. Patients were randomized to one of four treatment groups: standard-dose CsA (150–300 ng/ml for 3 months, followed by 100–200 ng/ml), MPA, and prednisone versus a regimen that included daclizumab induction, MPA, and prednisone in addition to either low-dose TAC (3–7 ng/ml), low-dose sirolimus (4–8 ng/ml), or low-dose CsA (50–100 ng/ml). The mean calculated glomerular filtration rate (GFR) at 12 months was highest in the TAC group (65.4 ml/minute) versus the other groups (56.7- 59.4 ml/min) and BPAR was lowest in the TAC group (12.3%) versus the other groups (24–37.2%). Allograft survival rate was also significantly higher in the TAC group (94.2%) versus the other groups (89.3–93.1%) (p = 0.02). Serious adverse events were most common in the sirolimus group (53.2%) versus the other groups (43.4–44.3%) [37]. Observational results at 3-year follow-up showed that the low-dose TAC group continued to have the highest GFR (68.6 ml/minute) compared to the other groups (65.3–68.6 ml/minute) [38]. The TAC group also continued to have the lowest BPAR rate and the highest rate of graft survival, although differences between the groups were reduced over time. Based on these analyses, complete CNI avoidance is not a recommended regimen at this time, and the authors concluded that low-dose TAC is the most beneficial and efficacious regimen, potentially avoiding negative effects on renal function [38].

Due to the fact that the results did not favor de novo CNI avoidance, the CsA Avoidance Eliminates Serious Adverse Renal Toxicity (CAESAR) trial investigated the efficacy and safety of de novo reduction and withdrawal of

CsA [39]. This prospective multicentered trial randomized 536 patients into three groups: standard-dose CsA, MPA, and prednisone versus daclizumab induction therapy with either low-dose CsA (50–100 ng/ml), MPA, and prednisone or low-dose CsA (withdrawn at 6 months), MPA, and prednisone. There was no difference between the three groups in terms of 12-month mean GFR, but the incidence of BPAR at 12 months was significantly higher in the CsA-withdrawal group (38 versus 25.4–27.5%) (p < 0.05). Therefore, the authors concluded that because improved renal function was not observed despite lower CNI exposure with CsA withdrawal and the incidence of BPAR was significantly higher—which could potentially damage organ function—a continuous low-dose CsA regimen should be recommended [39].

A recent meta-analysis including 19 trials and a total of 3321 patients evaluated three subgroups: de novo CNI minimization, elective CNI minimization and withdrawal (2 months post-transplant), and CNI minimization and withdrawal in declining renal function [40]. Improved GFR (4.4 ml/minute higher than controls, 95% CI 2.9–5.9) was apparent among all CNI-minimization trials, which may potentially impact long-term graft survival. Increased risk of BPAR was seen with elective CNI-withdrawal regimens, although this increase was not observed in CNI minimization for any subgroup or CNI withdrawal in the setting of renal dysfunction [40].

Overall, although CNI withdrawal may provide lower acute rejection rates than CNI avoidance, withdrawal should be carried out carefully and slowly in order to minimize the risk of rejection. Furthermore, in an attempt to balance the increased rate of BPAR with improved renal function, refining patient selection to identify a low-immunological-risk population that may benefit from this regimen is necessary. Although it is suggested that CNI minimization and withdrawal may be a safe alternative for patients with declining renal function, the additional benefit of stabilizing or improving renal function with late withdrawal is questionable, due to irreversible kidney tissue damage that may have already occurred prior to CNI discontinuation. In conclusion, de novo CNI dose reduction may be the most optimal regimen for sparing renal function and maintaining acceptable rejection rates, but long-term data are still needed to confirm that the short-term benefits seen with current trials will persist.

In the USA, the use of CsA has steadily declined since the introduction of TAC, based on the data described in this section [25]. In the UK, NICE recommends that the initial choice of TAC or CsA should be based on the potential impact of their related adverse events in individual transplant recipients [26].

ToR inhibitors
Pharmacology
Sirolimus and everolimus are macrolide derivatives that inhibit lymphocyte activation and proliferation [1,28,41–43]. Intracellularly, these agents complex with FKBP-12, subsequently binding to and modulating the activity of the ToR, which is a key regulatory kinase in cytokine-dependent T-cell proliferation. Inhibition of ToR results in the arrest of the cell-division cycle

in the G_1-to-S phase. Both ToR inhibitors also affect hematopoietic and nonhematopoietic cells [41–43].

Pharmaceutics and dosing

Sirolimus doses vary depending on its approved indication. In RTRs at low–moderate immunological risk, a loading dose of 6 mg should be given, followed by 2 mg/day maintenance [41,42]. Sirolimus is also indicated for use in RTRs at high immunological risk, defined as patients of African descent and/or those with previous RTRs where the graft was lost secondary to immunological reasons and/or those with high panel-reactive antibody (peak level >80%). In this population, a sirolimus loading dose of 15 mg is recommended, followed by a maintenance dose of 5 mg/day [41,42]. Everolimus is only indicated for prevention of rejection in low–moderate-risk RTRs when given in conjunction with basiliximab induction, reduced-dose CsA, and corticosteroids [41,43]. The recommended starting dose of everolimus is 0.75 mg twice daily, without the need for a loading dose.

Therapeutic drug monitoring

There is excellent correlation between whole-blood C_0 and the AUC for the ToR inhibitors [44]. Literature supports sirolimus C_0 ranges from 5 to 24 ng/ml, depending on institution-specific protocols [41,42,44]. The manufacturer has recommended goal C_0 in specific populations: in low–moderate-immunological-risk patients where CsA is withdrawn, the manufacturer recommends sirolimus C_0 be kept in the range of 16–24 ng/ml within 12 months [41]—thereafter, sirolimus C_0 should be 12–20 ng/ml; in high-immunological-risk patients, sirolimus C_0 should be within the range of 10–15 ng/ml. It should be noted that sirolimus has a half-life of approximately 62 hours. Utilization of the loading dose allows steady state to be achieved within 24–48 hours. However, in maintenance patients requiring dose adjustments, a new steady state will not be achieved for at least three half-lives, or 186 hours. In this situation, C_0 should be monitored 5–7 days after the dosage adjustment. For everolimus, the recommended C_0 goal is 3–8 ng/ml [41,43]. With a significantly shorter half-life, everolimus steady state can be reached with 90–150 hours.

Adverse events

The more frequently reported adverse events with the ToR inhibitors include myelosuppression, GI distress, headache, insomnia, arthralgias, tremor, hyperlipidemia, and rash [41]. Sirolimus' post-transplant complications, particularly the potential to prolong DGF—along with delayed wound healing, lymphocele formation, pneumonitis, and mucositis—have limited its de novo use [42]. Everolimus is indicated for de novo use despite the potential for a similar toxicity profile. Proteinuria and glomerulonephropathy have been reported with the ToR inhibitors, especially after conversion from a CNI [45–50]. Other important, yet rare, adverse events with these agents include hemolytic uremic syndrome/thrombotic microangiopathy and liver dysfunction [42].

Comparative efficacy

Early sirolimus studies focused on its use as an adjunct agent in combination with CsA and found a higher incidence of impaired renal function [51]. Newer studies have focused on its use as a primary immunosuppressant in lieu of the CNIs. The clinical use of sirolimus has been investigated in de novo transplantation with CNI avoidance regimens and CNI conversion protocols. Flechner and colleagues studied the de novo use of sirolimus with basiliximab induction therapy, MPA, and prednisone. Compared to a CsA arm, renal function was significantly better at 1, 2, and 5 years, with low acute rejection rates of approximately 10% [52–54]. Several trials emphasized the importance of having sirolimus C_0 of at least 10–15 ng/mL for the first 6 months, and this was evident in the SYMPHONY trial, in which the sirolimus group (target $C_0 = 4-8$ ng/ml) resulted in the highest rates of BPAR, compared to the other groups [37,55]. Several retrospective analyses have found sirolimus-based regimens to be associated with significantly worse long-term allograft survival. The largest of these studies was a retrospective analysis of the Scientific Registry of Renal Transplant Recipients that included over 2000 patients receiving immunosuppression with sirolimus and MPA [56]. In comparison to several other immunosuppressive regimens, the combination of sirolimus and MPA was associated with a higher 6-month BPAR rate (16 versus 11.2%; $p < 0.01$) and the lowest rate of allograft survival. For deceased-donor RTR, DGF was highest among the sirolimus and MPA group (47 versus 27%; $p < 0.001$). Furthermore, in a subgroup analysis of patients who were continued on the regimen at 6 months, conditional graft-survival rates were still the lowest among all the immunosuppressive regimens at 5 years post-transplant (64 versus 78%; $p = 0.001$) [56].

Due to inconclusive results and an increased incidence of DGF with de novo sirolimus regimens, recent studies have evaluated newer regimens that entail early (3–6 months post-transplant) and late (>6 months post-transplant) CNI withdrawal and conversion to sirolimus. The Spare the Nephron trial included 305 patients with standard triple-drug immunosuppression, who were randomized to either maintain their standard regimen or convert their CNI to sirolimus ($C_0 = 5-10$ ng/ml) at between 30 and 180 days post-transplant [57]. At 2 years post-conversion, GFR was significantly better in the sirolimus group compared to the CNI group ($p = 0.05$) and there was no difference in patient and graft survival or BPAR. Several randomized trial have evaluated late conversion of sirolimus in the setting of CNI toxicity or the development of chronic allograft nephropathy. The CONVERT trial randomized 830 CNI-based RTRs to maintain the standard regimen or convert to sirolimus ($C_0 = 8-20$ ng/ml) at between 6 and 120 months post-transplant [58]. Investigators demonstrated that patients with GFR >40 ml/minute and urine protein-to-creatinine ratio <0.11 at the time of conversion had significantly higher GFR (62.6 versus 59.9 ml/minute; $p = 0.009$) while maintaining a low incidence of BPAR (7.8%) after conversion. However, the investigators halted enrollment of patients with GFR 20–40 ml/minute due to an increased incidence of death and adverse events. Therefore, it is noted from this study that the timing of sirolimus conversion is crucial and that sirolimus conversion may be most beneficial prior to the deterioration of kidney function [58].

As for everolimus, several key phase-II and -III studies have demonstrated its efficacy and safety when used with a CsA-sparing regimen in de novo RTRs [43,59]. These studies also demonstrated that the use of everolimus with reduced-dose CsA allows for preservation of renal function without loss of efficacy, in comparison to full-dose CsA regimens [43,59].

In addition to the renal-sparing properties of the ToR inhibitors, there is increasing evidence that these agents also inhibit angiogenesis and vascular endothelial growth factor, thus preventing cancer development or slowing cancer-cell proliferation, particularly in skin cancers, lymphoma, and renal-cell carcinoma [43]. Although those trials will not be discussed in this review, sirolimus and everolimus may be considered in patients at high risk of cancer post-transplant and de novo cancer in the post-transplant setting [43].

Overall, further analysis is needed to identify the exact patient populations that will most benefit from the ToR inhibitors, and to determine the beneficial impact of long-term patient and graft survival. To date, sirolimus and everolimus have not been studied head to head, and the true clinical differences between the two agents are not known. Currently, NICE recommends that ToR inhibitors should be an option as part of an immunosuppressive regimen only in cases of proven intolerance to CNIs which necessitate complete withdrawal of this treatment [26].

Antiproliferatives

The antiproliferatives are generally considered adjuvant agents to be coadministered with a CNI [1,27]. The primary agents included in this class are AZA and the MPA derivatives, although other antiproliferatives, such as cyclophosphamide and leflunomide, have been used in transplantation.

Pharmacology

AZA is a prodrug for 6-mercaptopurine (6-MP), a purine analog [1,28,41]. 6-MP is incorporated into the cellular DNA, where it alters the synthesis and function of RNA, with a subsequent reduction in T-cell proliferation. MPA inhibits inosine monophosphate phosphate dehydrogenase (IMPDH), a key enzyme in the de novo pathway of guanosine nucleotide synthesis. IMPDH inhibition prevents the proliferation of cells that are dependent upon the de novo pathway for purine synthesis, including lymphocytes. Other cell lines are capable of purine synthesis via the salvage pathway, which MPA does not affect [1,28,41,60].

Pharmaceutics and dosing

Over the past 2 decades, AZA use has declined markedly, due in large part to the success of regimens containing MPA. MMF is a prodrug that is rapidly hydrolyzed to MPA following its oral absorption [1,28,41,60]. Enteric-coated MPA is absorbed in the intestine as the active moiety.

AZA is available in oral and IV formulations [41]. The typical oral dose of AZA is 1–2 mg/kg/day. The bioavailability of AZA is approximately 50%; therefore, the appropriate conversion of IV to oral dosing would be a doubling of the dose. Dose reductions in severely impaired renal function may be necessary due to accumulation of 6-MP and its metabolites [41].

MMF is available in capsules, tablets, an oral suspension, and as an injectable [41]. The recommended starting dose of MMF in RTRs is 2000 mg/day in two divided doses. The oral bioavailability of MMF exceeds 90%; therefore, conversion between oral and IV MMF is 1 : 1. Food may reduce the maximum concentration of MPA by up to 40%. However, the extent of MPA absorption is not affected by food, indicating that MMF may be administered with or without food [1,28,41].

Enteric-coated MPA is available in tablets [41]. The recommended starting dose of enteric-coated MPA is 720 mg twice daily. This dose provides equimolar MPA concentrations, seen with MMF 1000 mg twice daily [41,60]. Converting between the two MPA preparations is safe [60]. Administration of enteric-coated MPA can also be done without regards to food [41].

Adverse events

Myelosuppression is the most common adverse event of AZA. It is a dose-dependent and dose-limiting complication that often necessitates dose reductions [41]. Hepatotoxicity and GI distress have also been associated with AZA use. Importantly, pancreatitis and veno-occlusive disease of the liver have rarely ($<1\%$) been reported in patients on chronic AZA therapy [41].

The MPA derivatives have outstanding tolerability, with the most common adverse events being GI distress (both upper- and lower-GI-tract symptoms) and myelosuppression [41,60,61]. Enteric-coated MPA was developed in order to improve the upper-GI adverse-event profile seen with MMF [60]. In de novo and stable RTRs, the efficacy and tolerability outcomes are comparable with the two MPA derivatives [62,63]. There are no significant differences between GI side effects seen with the two formulations [60,64,65].

Therapeutic drug monitoring

TDM for AZA is not recommended. The exact role of MPA TDM is uncertain as there are conflicting results regarding actual improvement in efficacy and safety outcomes when using TDM. MPA AUC, but not C_0, has shown good correlation with efficacy in patients who are also receiving nondepleting-protein induction therapy and CsA [66–68]. Recently, three large randomized prospective trials have tried to address the role of TDM for MPA. The Adaption de Posologie du MMF en Greffe Renale (APOMYGRE) study showed that the prevalence of treatment failures was significantly lower in the TDM-dosed arm compared to the fixed-dose arm (29.2 versus 47.7%; $p = 0.03$) [69]. In contrast, the Fixed Dose versus Concentration Control (FDCC) study by van Gelder *et al.*, which had virtually identical study design and primary endpoint, did not show any differences in incidence of treatment failure or BPAR [68]. The differences in outcome between the two large trials may have been most influenced by the different methods used to calculate TDM for MPA.

Recently, the Opticept trial evaluated the safety and efficacy of MPA TDM in patients receiving TAC therapy [70]. The results of this trial suggest that TDM for MPA may be suitable in CNI-minimization regimens. However, it is inconclusive whether the low-dose CNI or TDM-dosed MPA was the influential factor driving the positive outcome of this trial. Overall, the use of MPA TDM in RTRs is not routinely recommended [71].

Comparative efficacy
The MPA derivatives have largely replaced AZA as the antiproliferative agent of choice in most renal-transplant centers. Most of the initial studies comparing MMF to AZA showed superior BPAR rates with MPA in combination with the nonmodified CsA formulation.

A recent systematic review including 19 trials and over 3100 patients was conducted to investigate whether MPA had greater efficacy than AZA [72]. The use of MPA significantly reduced risk of BPAR in combination with any CNI (RR 0.62, 95% CI 0.55–0.87; p < 0.00001), and graft loss was also significantly reduced in the MPA group compared to AZA (HR 0.76, 95% CI 0.59–0.98; p = 0.037). However, there were no significant differences in terms of patient survival, allograft function, CMV infection, hematological toxicities, or malignancy, although a greater incidence of diarrhea was seen in the MPA-treated patients. Therefore, the authors concluded that MPA should be used as first-line immunosuppression, given the reduction in risk of BPAR, and it may still be cost-effective when considering the overall treatment cost for BPAR and overall graft loss [72].

Co-Stimulation Blockade
Pharmacology
Belatacept binds to the CD80 and CD86 ligands, found on APCs. The CD80 and CD86 proteins are responsible for stimulating CD28 on inactive T-cells, an essential costimulatory interaction. Blockade of this co-stimulatory pathway results in T-cell anergy [73].

Pharmaceutics and Dosing
The recommended dosing regimen for belatacept is 10 mg/kg on the first day of transplantation, followed by an additional dose four days post-transplant, and again at the end of weeks 2, 4, 8, and 12, post-transplant. Beginning at the end of week 16 post-transplant, belatacept is dosed at 5 mg/kg and every four weeks thereafter. Belatacept requires access to an infusion-center, a hired home infusion service, or an infusion suite to ensure appropriate IV administration [73].

Adverse Events
The most common adverse effects associated with belatacept are infectious (urinary tract infection, 37%; upper respiratory infection, 15%), GI (diarrhea, 39%; constipation, 33%; nausea, 24%, vomiting, 22%), metabolic (hyperkalemia, 20%; hypokalemia 21%), and central nervous system (CNS; headache, 21%) complications. Other adverse effects include peripheral

edema, anemia, leukopenia, hypotension, arthralgia, and insomnia. Belatacept has a black-box warning for increased risk of developing post-transplant lymphoproliferative disorders (PTLD), especially in the CNS. Due to this risk, it is recommended that belatacept only be used in patients who present with a proven pre-existing immunity to Epstein-Barr virus (EBV) [73].

Comparative Efficacy

In a three-year, randomized, controlled, partially blinded, parallel group, multicenter study, treatment with two belatacept-based regimens was compared to a cyclosporine-based regimen evaluating three co-primary outcomes: a composite patient and graft survival, composite renal impairment endpoint and the incidence of BPAR at 12 months [74]. All patients received basiliximab induction and maintenance therapy with MMF and corticosteroids. Patients were randomized in a 1:1:1 fashion to one of two different belatacept-based regimens or CsA.

Both belatacept regimens met the non-inferiority margin of 10% as well as a more rigorous threshold of 5% for the co-primary endpoint of patient and graft survival compared to the CsA group. Evaluation of the co-primary composite renal impairment endpoint demonstrated that renal function was superior in patients who were randomized to belatacept versus cyclosporine. The incidence of BPAR at 12 months was 22% in the higher-dose belatacept group, 17% in the lower-dose belatacept group, and 7% in the cyclosporine group. The lower-dose belatacept group was deemed non-inferior for preventing BPAR compared to the CsA by satisfying a 20% margin for comparison. The mean measured GFR was 13–15 mL/min higher in the belatacept group despite a higher incidence of BPAR. Cardiovascular and metabolic outcomes were considerably better in both belatacept groups compared to CsA. No differences were noted in the incidence of the most frequent adverse events (anemia, UTI, hypertension, constipation, diarrhea, and nausea) between treatment groups [74].

Corticosteroids

Pharmacology

Corticosteroids have a multitude of therapeutic effects. Their exact immunosuppressive mechanism of action is not fully understood, but it is believed that they are an effective inhibitor of T-cell and APC-derived cytokine expression and dendritic cell function [1,28,41]. In a more nonspecific manner, corticosteroids cause general anti-inflammatory effects that may affect monocyte migration [1,28,41].

Pharmaceutics and dosing

The most commonly used corticosteroids in transplantation are methylprednisolone (IV and oral) and prednisone (oral), although prednisolone and dexamethasone have also been shown to be effective immunosuppressants [41]. There is no consensus on the optimal dose or maintenance schedule of steroids following renal transplantation. Corticosteroid doses vary according to center-specific protocols and patient characteristics. A typical regime might include a bolus of IV methylprednisolone 100–500 mg

Table 10.4 Common adverse events associated with corticosteroids [1,7,28].

Body system	Adverse event
Cardiovascular	Hyperlipidemia, hypertension
Central nervous system	Anxiety, insomnia, mood changes, psychosis
Dermatological	Acne, diaphoresis, ecchymosis, hirsutism, impaired wound-healing, petechiae, thin skin
Endocrine/metabolic	Cushing syndrome, hyperglycemia, sodium and water retention
Gastrointestinal	Gastritis, increased appetite, nausea, vomiting, diarrhea, peptic ulcers
Hematological	Leukocytosis
Neuromuscular/skeletal	Arthralgia, impaired growth, osteoporosis, skeletal muscle weakness
Ocular	Cataracts, glaucoma
Respiratory	Epistaxis

at the time of transplant, tapered over several days to a maintenance dose of prednisone 20 mg/day. Further dose reductions occur over subsequent weeks and months post-transplant. Doses of 2.5–5.0 mg/day are commonly used for long-term maintenance therapy.

Adverse events

Corticosteroids are associated with a variety of acute and chronic toxicities, including osteoporosis, hyperlipidemia, hypertension, insulin resistance, diabetes, cataracts, poor wound-healing, and growth retardation (Table 10.4). One analysis estimated the cost of corticosteroid-related adverse events to be $5300 (1996 US dollars) per patient per year [73]. A long-term survival analysis by Ojo *et al.* evaluating over 18 000 patients revealed that death with a functioning graft accounted for 40% of all graft loss and that the leading cause of death was cardiovascular disease [74]. There has thus been strong incentive to investigate protocols that focus on corticosteroid-sparing or -avoidance in order to balance the long-term cardiovascular side effects associated with corticosteroids without compromising long-term graft survival.

Steroid-minimization protocols

Steroid withdrawal

In an attempt to minimize steroid-related side effects, many studies have investigated several approaches to steroid withdrawal, including early withdrawal (within 1–3 weeks post-transplant), late withdrawal (after the first 6 months), and complete avoidance (within 7 days). Recently, the practice of early steroid withdrawal (ESW), typically defined as the cessation of steroids within the first 7 days of transplantation, has gained merit. Vincenti and colleagues performed an open-label analysis of 337 patients randomized with a 1 : 1 : 1 ratio to three different treatment arms [75]. Each patient received the IL-2 receptor antagonist basiliximab for induction therapy and both modified CsA and enteric-coated MPA as maintenance immunosuppression. The three treatment arms included no IV or oral steroids at any time (steroid avoidance), withdrawal from steroids at postoperative day 7 (steroid withdrawal), and patients who received long-term maintenance corticosteroid therapy. It was shown that a large percentage of patients in the steroid-avoidance group required add-on steroid therapy at some point during follow-up in order to maintain appropriate graft function. However, patients who received ESW had comparable rejection rates to the standard steroid-maintenance group, and a more favorable metabolic profile [75]. A similar analysis comparing two arms—ESW and a standard maintenance steroid protocol—found that there was a slightly increased risk of biopsy-proven BPAR in the ESW group, specifically steroid-responsive Banff 1A, but a significantly improved metabolic outcome. However, the two groups had similar 1-year allograft survival and patient outcomes [76]. Review of the literature in two large meta-analyses found that RTRs who were considered to have a low immunological risk for rejection and graft loss had similar rates of BPAR and allograft survival compared to patients who were maintained on corticosteroids for immunosuppression [77,78]. The majority of concerns about ESW address the lack of long-term outcomes, although a recent large, retrospective analysis suggests that the use of ESW versus standard maintenance steroids results in comparable allograft survival [79].

Treatment of acute rejection

The key to the effective management of BPAR is an accurate and timely diagnosis and the prompt administration of potent immunosuppression. Ideally, a balance must be struck between reversing the rejection episode and limiting excessive impairment of the host defenses. Currently, corticosteroids and rATG are the main components of antirejection therapy.

Corticosteroids
High-dose corticosteroids have been the mainstay of acute cellular rejection therapy since the inception of their use in transplantation. Oral corticosteroids (rejection reversal rates of 56–72%) have been successfully employed for the treatment of acute rejection, but IV methylprednisolone (rejection reversal rates of 60–76%) remains the treatment of choice [80,81]. Pulse-dose methylprednisolone therapy consists of the administration of 250–1000 mg/day for 3–4 days. One study demonstrated that the high doses were associated with a greater improvement in renal function, while the lower doses were linked to a lower prevalence of infectious complications [82].

Antithymocyte globulins
The ATG agents have been shown to successfully reverse more than 90% of acute rejection episodes [83]. In comparison with the corticosteroids, the use of ATG preparations for treatment of acute rejection has resulted in a more rapid reversal of rejection, fewer repeat rejection episodes, and

better long-term graft survival [83,84]. A study by Gaber *et al.* evaluated rATG and eATG for the treatment of acute rejection in RTRs [85]. Patients received a 7–14 day course of either rATG (1.5 mg/kg/day; n = 82) or eATG (15 mg/kg/day; n = 81), which was initiated within a day of BPAR. The successful response rate for rATG was significantly greater than that for eATG (rATG = 87.8%; eATG = 76.3%). rATG was found to increase the duration of subsequent rejection-free graft survival for those who successfully achieved initial response (p = 0.011). Adverse-event rates were similar in both groups [85].

Future immunosuppressive agents

The immunosuppressant armamentarium is expanding, with novel small molecules and biological agents currently in clinical development [86].

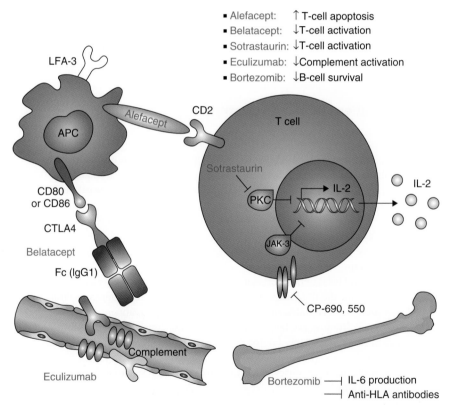

Figure 10.2 JAK3 inhibitor (CP-690,550), PKC inhibitor (sotrastaurin), and CD28 inhibitor (belatacept) inhibit T-cell activation, whereas LFA-3–Ig depletes allogenic T-cells. Bortezomib impairs plasma-cell production of anti-HLA antibodies and eculizumab inhibits complement activation mediated by anti-HLA antibodies. APC, antigen-presenting cell; IL, interleukin; JAK-3, Janus kinase 3; LFA-3, lymphocyte-function-associated antigen-3; PKC, protein kinase C. (Reproduced by permission from Macmillan Publishers Ltd: from [87] Durrbach *et al.* Advances in immunosuppression for renal transplantation. *Nat Rev Nephrol* 2010;6:160–7)

These newer agents appear promising and may represent the emergence of novel immunosuppressive agents that can deliver immunosuppression with little long-term toxicity. Figure 10.2 schematically depicts the mechanisms of action of these potential future immunosuppressive agents. A brief review of these agents is given in this section.

Alefacept

Alefacept is a fusion protein that binds to CD2 and inhibits activation of T-lymphocytes [87]. A renal-transplant study in nonhuman primates found that alefacept, when combined with CTLA-4-IgG and sirolimus, significantly improved allograft survival [88]. A study is ongoing to assess the efficacy and safety of this agent in RTRs [89].

Bortezomib

Bortozemib is a 26S proteosome inhibitor that disrupts cellular homeostasis and induces cell death [87]. This agent is approved for use in myeloma. Several case reports and small-scale studies (presented in abstract form only) suggest that it may be useful in the management of pretransplant, highly sensitized patients and for treatment of antibody-mediated rejection (AMR) [90,91]. Additional studies with rigorous immunological follow-up are required before recommendations can be made for the routine use of this agent.

Eculizimab

Eculizimab is a monoclonal antibody that inhibits complement protein C5 cleavage into C5a and C5b and subsequently inhibits the formation of the membrane attack complex [87]. This agent is licensed for the treatment of paroxysmal nocturnal hemoglobinuria. Due to its ability to blunt the complement cascade, it has been used for the treatment of AMR, as well as for the post-transplant management of hemolytic–uremic syndrome [92,93]. Clinical trials are ongoing and positive results are required before the routine use of this medication can be recommended [94,95].

Rituximab

Rituximab is an anti-CD20 humanized, monoclonal antibody that is licensed for use in CD20-positive non-Hodgkin lymphoma, chronic lymphoid leukemia, and rheumatoid arthritis [41]. CD20 is a surface antigen expressed on all circulating, mature B-cells. Due to its anti-B-cell properties, it has been used in pretransplant desensitization protocols, as well as for the treatment of AMR [96,97]. Another area in which rituximab has shown great promise is ABO-incompatible kidney transplantation. In a study by Fuchinoue *et al.*, rituximab, when given as part of a preoperative regimen in ABO-incompatible transplant recipients, yielded even better renal function than is found in ABO-compatible patients not receiving this agent [98]. This benefit was seen without an increase in toxicities. There has also been a recent shift in focus on B-cells and their ability to contribute to acute cellular rejection due to their ability to echo the effect of APCs. The ability of rituximab to deplete a patient of circulating mature B-cells led Tyden and colleagues to test its use as a single-dose induction agent in RTRs in a prospective, randomized, double-blind, placebo-controlled multicenter study [99]. In this analysis, rituximab showed no improvements in transplant-related outcomes. At this time, the use of rituximab as sole induction agent for renal transplantation is questionable, especially given the data showing no benefit versus placebo [99].

Sotrastaurin (AEB071)

Sotrastaurin is a novel oral immunosuppressant that prevents T-lymphocyte activation through inhibition of protein kinase C [87]. An animal study has shown prolonged renal allograft survival with sotrastaurin use. It is currently in phase II of clinical development as a maintenance immunosuppressant following renal transplant [87,100]. In the initial published clinical trial, sotrastaurin appeared to have good efficacy and tolerability when coadministered with TAC, but it seems to provide inadequate immunosuppression in a CNI-withdrawal regimen [101]. Longer-term evaluation of sotrastaurin with TAC is currently ongoing [102].

Tofacitinib (CP690550)

Tofacitinib, formerly known as tasocitinib, is an oral inhibitor of Janus kinase 3, which reduces natural-killer and T-lymphocyte subsets [87]. A randomized pilot study evaluated two different doses of tofacitinib (30 and 60 mg/day) versus TAC in de novo RTRs [103]. The low-dose tofacitinib group had a similar efficacy and tolerability profile to the TAC group. The higher dose of tofacitinib was associated with a higher rate of CMV and BK virus infection [103].

Voclosporin (ISA247)

Voclosporin, a CsA analog, is a new-generation CNI with reduced nephrotoxicity [104]. In its phase-II clinical trial, voclosporin showed similar efficacy to TAC following renal transplantation. It appears to have a safety benefit compared to TAC in terms of new-onset diabetes, triglycerides, magnesium, and neurological adverse events [104].

References

1 Halloran PF. Immunosuppressive drugs for kidney transplantation. *N Engl J Med* 2004;351:2715–2729.
2 Gabardi S, Martin ST, Roberts KL, Grafals M. Induction immunosuppressive therapies in renal transplantation. *Am J Health Syst Pharm* 2011;68:211–218.
3 Larsen CP, Knechtle SJ, Adams A, Pearson T, and Kirk AD. A new look at blockade of T-cell costimulation: a therapeutic strategy for long-term maintenance immunosuppression. *Am J Transplant* 2006;6(5):876–883.
4 Hardinger KL. Rabbit antithymocyte globulin induction therapy in adult renal transplantation. *Pharmacotherapy* 2006;26:1771–1783.
5 Nashan B. Antibody induction therapy in renal transplant patients receiving calcineurin-inhibitor immunosuppressive regimens: a comparative review. *BioDrugs* 2005;19:39–46.
6 Food and Drug Administration. Important drug information. Available from http://www.fda.gov/downloads/Drugs/DrugSafety/DrugShortages/UCM 194907.pdf (accessed April 9, 2011).

7 Micromedex Healthcare Series. Greenwood Village, CO: Thomson Healthcare; 2007.

8 Ramirez CB, Marino IR. The role of basiliximab induction therapy in organ transplantation. *Expert Opin Biol Ther* 2007;7:137–148.

9 Andreoni KA, Brayman KL, Guidinger MK, Sommers CM, Sung RS. Kidney and pancreas transplantation in the United States, 1996–2005. *Am J Transplant* 2007;7:1359.

10 Nashan B, Moore R, Amlot P, Schmidt AG, Abeywickrama K, Soulillou JP. Randomised trial of basiliximab versus placebo for control of acute cellular rejection in renal allograft recipients. CHIB 201 International Study Group. *Lancet* 1997;350:1193–1198.

11 Webster AC, Ruster LP, McGee R, *et al.* Interleukin 2 receptor antagonists for kidney transplant recipients. *Cochrane Database Syst Rev*:CD003897.

12 Kirk AD. Induction immunosuppression. *Transplantation* 2006;82:593–602.

13 Beiras-Fernandez A, Thein E, Hammer C. Induction of immunosuppression with polyclonal antithymocyte globulins: an overview. *Exp Clin Transplant* 2003;1:79–84.

14 Lopez M, Clarkson MR, Albin M, Sayegh MH, Najafian N. A novel mechanism of action for anti-thymocyte globulin: induction of CD4+CD25 +Foxp3+ regulatory T cells. *J Am Soc Nephrol* 2006;17:2844–853.

15 Goggins WC, Pascual MA, Powelson JA, *et al.* A prospective, randomized, clinical trial of intraoperative versus postoperative thymoglobulin in adult cadaveric renal transplant recipients. *Transplantation* 2003;76:798–802.

16 Lo A, Olson B, Gaber L, Gaber A. Thymoglobulin for Induction and for Treatment of Rejection in Renal Transplant Recipients (abstract). Washington, DC: American Transplant Congress; 2003.

17 Guttmann RD, Flemming C. Sequential biological immunosuppression. Induction therapy with rabbit antithymocyte globulin. *Clin Transplant* 1997;11:185–192.

18 Brennan DC, Flavin K, Lowell JA, *et al.* A randomized, double-blinded comparison of Thymoglobulin versus Atgam for induction immunosuppressive therapy in adult renal transplant recipients. *Transplantation* 1999;67: 1011–1018.

19 Hardinger KL, Rhee S, Buchanan P, *et al.* A prospective, randomized, double-blinded comparison of thymoglobulin versus Atgam for induction immunosuppressive therapy: 10-year results. *Transplantation* 2008;86: 947–952.

20 Brennan DC, Daller JA, Lake KD, Cibrik D, Del Castillo D. Rabbit antithymocyte globulin versus basiliximab in renal transplantation. *N Engl J Med* 2006;355:1967–1977.

21 Morris PJ, Russell NK. Alemtuzumab (Campath-1H): a systematic review in organ transplantation. *Transplantation* 2006;81:1361–1367.

22 Ciancio G, Burke GW, 3rd,. Alemtuzumab (Campath-1H) in kidney transplantation. *Am J Transplant* 2008;8:15–20.

23 Jones JL, Phuah CL, Cox AL, *et al.* IL-21 drives secondary autoimmunity in patients with multiple sclerosis, following therapeutic lymphocyte depletion with alemtuzumab (Campath-1H). *J Clin Invest* 2009;119:2052–2061.

24 Hanaway MJ, Woodle ES, Mulgaonkar S, *et al.* Alemtuzumab induction in renal transplantation. *N Engl J Med* 2011;364:1909–19.

25 Andreoni KA, Brayman KL, Guidinger MK, Sommers CM, Sung RS. Kidney and pancreas transplantation in the United States, 1996–2005. *Am J Transplant* 2007;7:1359–1375.

26 National Institute for Health and Clinical Excellence. Immunosuppressive therapy for renal transplantation in adults. Available from http://www.nice .org.uk/nicemedia/live/11544/32940/32940.pdf (accessed April 9, 2011).

27 Norman DJ, Turka LA. Primer on Transplantation, 2nd ed. Mt Laurel, NJ/Malden, MA: American Society of Transplantation/Blackwell Publising; 2001.

28 Hardinger KL, Koch MJ, Brennan DC. Current and future immunosuppressive strategies in renal transplantation. *Pharmacotherapy* 2004;24:1159–1176.

29 Perner F. Cyclosporine microemulsion (Neoral) absorption profiling and sparse-sample predictors during the first 3 months after renal transplantation. *Am J Transplant* 2002;2:148–156.

30 Reams BD, Palmer SM. Sublingual tacrolimus for immunosuppression in lung transplantation: a potentially important therapeutic option in cystic fibrosis. *Am J Respir Med* 2002;1:91–98.

31 Reams D, Rea J, Davis D, Palmer S. Utility of sublingual tacrolimus in cystic fibrosis patients after lung transplantation. *J Heart Lung Transplant* 2001; 20:207–208.

32 Walfe JA, McCann RL, Sanfilippo F. Cyclosporine-associated microangiopathy in renal transplantation: a severe but potentially reversible form of early graft injury. *Transplantation* 1986;41:541–544.

33 Myers BD. Cyclosporine nephrotoxicity. *Kidney Int* 1986;30:964–974.

34 Holman MJ, Gonwa TA, Cooper B, *et al.* FK506-associated thrombotic thrombocytopenic purpura. *Transplantation* 1993;55:205–206.

35 Trimarchi HM, Truong LD, Brennan S, Gonzalez JM, Suki WN. FK506-associated thrombotic microangiopathy: report of two cases and review of the literature. *Transplantation* 1999;67:539–544.

36 Webster AC, Woodroffe RC, Taylor RS, Chapman JR, Craig JC. Tacrolimus versus ciclosporin as primary immunosuppression for kidney transplant recipients: meta-analysis and meta-regression of randomised trial data. *BMJ* 2005;331:810.

37 Ekberg H, Tedesco-Silva H, Demirbas A, *et al.* Reduced exposure to calcineurin inhibitors in renal transplantation. *N Engl J Med* 2007;357: 2562–2575.

38 Ekberg H, Bernasconi C, Tedesco-Silva H, *et al.* Calcineurin inhibitor minimization in the Symphony study: observational results 3 years after transplantation. *Am J Transplant* 2009;9:1876–1885.

39 Ekberg H, Grinyo J, Nashan B, *et al.* Cyclosporine sparing with mycophenolate mofetil, daclizumab and corticosteroids in renal allograft recipients: the CAESAR Study. *Am J Transplant* 2007;7:560–570.

40 Moore J, Middleton L, Cockwell P, *et al.* Calcineurin inhibitor sparing with mycophenolate in kidney transplantation: a systematic review and meta-analysis. *Transplantation* 2009;87:591–605.

41 Micromedex Healthcare Series. Greenwood Village, CO: Thomson Healthcare; 2010.

42 Morath C, Arns W, Schwenger V, *et al.* Sirolimus in renal transplantation. *Nephrol Dial Transplant* 2007;22(Suppl 8):viii61–viii5.

43 Gabardi S, Baroletti SA. Everolimus: a proliferation signal inhibitor with clinical applications in organ transplantation, oncology, and cardiology. *Pharmacotherapy* 2010;30:1044–1056.

44 MacDonald A, Scarola J, Burke JT, Zimmerman JJ. Clinical pharmacokinetics and therapeutic drug monitoring of sirolimus. *Clin Ther* 2000;22(Suppl B):B101–B121.

45 Franco AF, Martini D, Abensur H, Noronha IL. Proteinuria in transplant patients associated with sirolimus. *Transplant Proc* 2007;39:449–452.

46 Pinheiro HS, Amaro TA, Braga AM, Bastos MG. Post-rapamycin proteinuria: incidence, evolution, and therapeutic handling at a single center. *Transplant Proc* 2006;38:3476–3478.

47 Rangan GK. Sirolimus-associated proteinuria and renal dysfunction. *Drug Saf* 2006;29:1153–1161.

48 Ruiz JC, Campistol JM, Sanchez-Fructuoso A, *et al.* Increase of proteinuria after conversion from calcineurin inhibitor to sirolimus-based treatment in kidney transplant patients with chronic allograft dysfunction. *Nephrol Dial Transplant* 2006;21:3252–3257.

49 van den Akker JM, Wetzels JF, Hoitsma AJ. Proteinuria following conversion from azathioprine to sirolimus in renal transplant recipients. *Kidney Int* 2006;70:1355–1357.

50 Letavernier E, Pe'raldi MN, Pariente A, Morelon E, Legendre C. Proteinuria following a switch from calcineurin inhibitors to sirolimus. *Transplantation* 2005;80:1198–1203.

51 Flechner SM. Sirolimus in kidney transplantation indications and practical guidelines: de novo sirolimus-based therapy without calcineurin inhibitors. *Transplantation* 2009;87:S1–S6.

52 Flechner SM, Goldfarb D, Modlin C, *et al.* Kidney transplantation without calcineurin inhibitor drugs: a prospective, randomized trial of sirolimus versus cyclosporine. *Transplantation* 2002;74:1070–1076.

53 Flechner SM, Kurian SM, Solez K, *et al.* De novo kidney transplantation without use of calcineurin inhibitors preserves renal structure and function at two years. *Am J Transplant* 2004;4:1776–1785.

54 Flechner SM, Goldfarb D, Solez K, *et al.* Kidney transplantation with sirolimus and mycophenolate mofetil-based immunosuppression: 5-year results of a randomized prospective trial compared to calcineurin inhibitor drugs. *Transplantation* 2007;83:883–892.

55 Webster AC, Lee VW, Chapman JR, Craig JC. Target of rapamycin inhibitors (sirolimus and everolimus) for primary immunosuppression of kidney transplant recipients: a systematic review and meta-analysis of randomized trials. *Transplantation* 2006;81:1234–1248.

56 Srinivas TR, Schold JD, Guerra G, Eagan A, Bucci CM, Meier-Kriesche HU. Mycophenolate mofetil/sirolimus compared to other common immunosuppressive regimens in kidney transplantation. *Am J Transplant* 2007;7:586–594.

57 Weir MR, Mulgaonkar S, Chan L, *et al.* Mycophenolate mofetil-based immunosuppression with sirolimus in renal transplantation: a randomized, controlled Spare-the-Nephron trial. *Kidney Int* 2011;79:897–907.

58 Schena FP, Pascoe MD, Alberu J, *et al.* Conversion from calcineurin inhibitors to sirolimus maintenance therapy in renal allograft recipients: 24-month efficacy and safety results from the CONVERT trial. *Transplantation* 2009;87:233–242.

59 Nashan B, Curtis J, Ponticelli C, Mourad G, Jaffe J, Haas T. Everolimus and reduced-exposure cyclosporine in de novo renal-transplant recipients: a three-year phase II, randomized, multicenter, open-label study. *Transplantation* 2004;78:1332–1340.

60 Gabardi S, Tran JL, Clarkson MR. Enteric-coated mycophenolate sodium. *Ann Pharmacother* 2003;37:1685–1693.

61 Hardinger KL, Brennan DC, Lowell J, Schnitzler MA. Long-term outcome of gastrointestinal complications in renal transplant patients treated with mycophenolate mofetil. *Transpl Int* 2004;17:609–616.

62 Budde K, Curtis J, Knoll G, *et al*. Enteric-coated mycophenolate sodium can be safely administered in maintenance renal transplant patients: results of a 1-year study. *Am J Transplant* 2004;4:237–243.

63 Salvadori M, Holzer H, de Mattos A, *et al*. Enteric-coated mycophenolate sodium is therapeutically equivalent to mycophenolate mofetil in de novo renal transplant patients. *Am J Transplant* 2004;4:231–236.

64 Budde K, Knoll G, Curtis J, *et al*. Long-term safety and efficacy after conversion of maintenance renal transplant recipients from mycophenolate mofetil (MMF) to enteric-coated mycophenolate sodium (EC-MPA, myfortic). *Clin Nephrol* 2006;66:103–111.

65 Salvadori M, Holzer H, Civati G, *et al*. Long-term administration of enteric-coated mycophenolate sodium (EC-MPS; myfortic) is safe in kidney transplant patients. *Clin Nephrol* 2006;66:112–119.

66 Shaw LM, Figurski M, Milone MC, Trofe J, Bloom RD. Therapeutic drug monitoring of mycophenolic acid. *Clin J Am Soc Nephrol* 2007;2:1062–1072.

67 van Gelder T. Mycophenolate blood level monitoring: recent progress. *Am J Transplant* 2009;9:1495–1499.

68 van Gelder T, Hilbrands LB, Vanrenterghem Y, *et al*. A randomized double-blind, multicenter plasma concentration controlled study of the safety and efficacy of oral mycophenolate mofetil for the prevention of acute rejection after kidney transplantation. *Transplantation* 1999;68:261–266.

69 Le Meur Y, Buchler M, Thierry A, *et al*. Individualized mycophenolate mofetil dosing based on drug exposure significantly improves patient outcomes after renal transplantation. *Am J Transplant* 2007;7:2496–2503.

70 Gaston RS, Kaplan B, Shah T, *et al*. Fixed- or controlled-dose mycophenolate mofetil with standard- or reduced-dose calcineurin inhibitors: the Opticept trial. *Am J Transplant* 2009;9:1607–1619.

71 Knight SR, Morris PJ. Does the evidence support the use of mycophenolate mofetil therapeutic drug monitoring in clinical practice? A systematic review. *Transplantation* 2008;85:1675–1685.

72 Knight SR, Russell NK, Barcena L, Morris PJ. Mycophenolate mofetil decreases acute rejection and may improve graft survival in renal transplant recipients when compared with azathioprine: a systematic review. *Transplantation* 2009;87:785–794.

73 Veenstra DL, Best JH, Hornberger J, Sullivan SD, Hricik DE. Incidence and long-term cost of steroid-related side effects after renal transplantation. *Am J Kidney Dis* 1999;33:829–839.

74 Ojo AO, Meier-Kriesche HU, Hanson JA, *et al*. Mycophenolate mofetil reduces late renal allograft loss independent of acute rejection. *Transplantation* 2000;69:2405–2409.

75 Vincenti F, Schena FP, Paraskevas S, Hauser IA, Walker RG, Grinyo J. A randomized, multicenter study of steroid avoidance, early steroid withdrawal or standard steroid therapy in kidney transplant recipients. *Am J Transplant* 2008;8:307–316.

76 Woodle ES, First MR, Pirsch J, Shihab F, Gaber AO, Van Veldhuisen P. A prospective, randomized, double-blind, placebo-controlled multicenter trial comparing early (7 day) corticosteroid cessation versus long-term, low-dose corticosteroid therapy. *Ann Surg* 2008;248:564–577.

77 Knight SR, Morris PJ. Steroid avoidance or withdrawal after renal transplantation increases the risk of acute rejection but decreases cardiovascular risk. *A meta-analysis. Transplantation* 2010;89:1–14.

78 Pascual J, Quereda C, Zamora J, Hernandez D. Updated metaanalysis of steroid withdrawal in renal transplant patients on calcineurin inhibitor and mycophenolate mofetil. *Transplant Proc* 2005;37:3746–3748.

79 Matas AJ, Gillingham K, Kandaswamy R, *et al*. Kidney transplant half-life (t[1/2]) after rapid discontinuation of prednisone. *Transplantation* 2009;87:100–102.

80 Mussche MM, Ringoir SM, Lameire NN. High intravenous doses of methylprednisolone for acute cadaveric renal allograft rejection. *Nephron* 1976;16:287–291.

81 Gray D, Shepherd H, Daar A, Oliver DO, Morris PJ. Oral versus intravenous high-dose steroid treatment of renal allograft rejection. The big shot or not? *Lancet* 1978;1:117–118.

82 Kauffman HM, Jr.,, Stromstad SA, Sampson D, Stawicki AT. Randomized steroid therapy of human kidney transplant rejection. *Transplant Proc* 1979;11:36–38.

83 Filo RS, Smith EJ, Leapman SB. Therapy of acute cadaveric renal allograft rejection with adjunctive antithymocyte globulin. *Transplantation* 1980;30:445–449.

84 Shield CF, 3rd,, Cosimi AB, Tolkoff-Rubin N, Rubin RH, Herrin J, Russell PS. Use of antithymocyte globulin for reversal of acute allograft rejection. *Transplantation* 1979;28:461–464.

85 Gaber AO, First MR, Tesi RJ, *et al*. Results of the double-blind, randomized, multicenter, phase III clinical trial of Thymoglobulin versus Atgam in the treatment of acute graft rejection episodes after renal transplantation. *Transplantation* 1998;66:29–37.

86 Yabu JM, Vincenti F. Novel immunosuppression: small molecules and biologics. *Semin Nephrol* 2007;27:479–486.

87 Durrbach A, Francois H, Beaudreuil S, Jacquet A, Charpentier B. Advances in immunosuppression for renal transplantation. *Nat Rev Nephrol* 2010;6:160–167.

88 Weaver TA, Charafeddine AH, Agarwal A, *et al*. Alefacept promotes co-stimulation blockade based allograft survival in nonhuman primates. *Nat Med* 2009;15:746–749.

89 ClinicalTrials.gov. A study to assess the safety and efficacy of alefacept in kidney transplant recipients. Available from http://clinicaltrials.gov/ct2/show /NCT00543569 (accessed April 9, 2011).

90 Flechner SM, Fatica R, Askar M, *et al*. The role of proteasome inhibition with bortezomib in the treatment of antibody-mediated rejection after kidney-only or kidney-combined organ transplantation. *Transplantation* 2010; 90:1486–1492.

91 Everly MJ, Everly JJ, Susskind B, *et al*. Bortezomib provides effective therapy for antibody- and cell-mediated acute rejection. *Transplantation* 2008;86:1754–1761.

92 Stegall MD, Gloor JM. Deciphering antibody-mediated rejection: new insights into mechanisms and treatment. *Curr Opin Organ Transplant* 2010;15:8–10.

93 Kavanagh D, Richards A, Goodship T, Jalanko H. Transplantation in atypical hemolytic uremic syndrome. *Semin Thromb Hemost* 2010;36:653–659.

94 ClinicalTrials.gov. Eculizumab therapy for chronic complement-mediated injury in kidney transplantation. Available from http://clinicaltrials.gov/ct2

/show/NCT01327573?term=eculizumab+and+renal+transplant&rank=5 (accessed April 9, 2011).

95 ClinicalTrials.gov. Eculizumab added to conventional treatment in the prevention of antibody-mediated rejection in ABO blood group incompatible living donor kidney transplantation. Available from http://clinicaltrials.gov /ct2/show/NCT01095887?term=eculizumab+and+renal+transplant& rank=3 (accessed April 9, 2011).

96 Vo AA, Lukovsky M, Toyoda M, *et al.* Rituximab and intravenous immune globulin for desensitization during renal transplantation. *N Engl J Med* 2008;359:242–251.

97 Jordan SC, Peng A, Vo AA. Therapeutic strategies in management of the highly HLA-sensitized and ABO-incompatible transplant recipients. *Contrib Nephrol* 2009;162:13–26.

98 Fuchinoue S, Ishii Y, Sawada T, *et al.* The 5-Year Outcome of ABO-Incompatible Kidney Transplantation With Rituximab Induction. *Transplantation* 2011;91:853–857.

99 Tyden G, Genberg H, Tollemar J, *et al.* A randomized, doubleblind, placebo-controlled, study of single-dose rituximab as induction in renal transplantation. *Transplantation* 2009;87:1325–1329.

100 Matz M, Naik M, Mashreghi MF, Glander P, Neumayer HH, Budde K. Evaluation of the novel protein kinase C inhibitor sotrastaurin as immunosuppressive therapy after renal transplantation. *Expert Opin Drug Metab Toxicol* 2011;7:103–113.

101 Budde K, Sommerer C, Becker T, *et al.* Sotrastaurin, a novel small molecule inhibiting protein kinase C: first clinical results in renal-transplant recipients. *Am J Transplant* 2010;10:571–581.

102 ClinicalTrials.gov. Efficacy, safety, tolerability, and pharmacokinetics of sotrastaurin combined with tacrolimus vs. a mycophenolic acid-tacrolimus regimen in renal transplant patients. http://clinicaltrials.gov/ct2/show/NCT 01064791?term=sotrastaurin+and+renal+transplant&rank=1 (accessed April 9, 2011).

103 Busque S, Leventhal J, Brennan DC, *et al.* Calcineurin-inhibitor-free immunosuppression based on the JAK inhibitor CP-690,550: a pilot study in de novo kidney allograft recipients. *Am J Transplant* 2009;9:1936–1945.

104 Cooper JE, Wiseman AC. Novel immunosuppressive agents in kidney transplantation. *Clin Nephrol* 2010;73:333–343.

11 Conclusion

Nizam Mamode[1] and Raja Kandaswamy[2]

[1]Guy's and St Thomas' Hospital, Great Ormond Street Hospital, UK
[2]Department of Surgery, University of Minnesota, USA

Transplantation has been one of the great success stories of the 20th century, and in our lifetimes has moved from an experimental technique—in the early years, often fraught with catastrophic complications—to a widely performed, often routine, procedure with excellent results. As we progress into the 21st century, the potential for further developments remains undiminished.

Currently, living donation is considered the best option for renal transplantation, with 1-year graft survival rates of about 98%. Paired-exchange schemes, nondirected (altruistic) donations, and extended chains are all ensuring that living-donation rates are increasing. Criteria for donor acceptance are widening—for example, with the use of obese or well-controlled hypertensive donors, or those with urolithiasis—but long-term data on such donors are needed to ensure safety. Antibody-incompatible programs are now increasingly common, and results from blood-group-incompatible renal transplants appear to be comparable with those from compatible living donors. Transplants are being offered to those who would previously have been denied an organ due to human leukocyte antigen (HLA) incompatibility. The newfound focus on antibody-mediated rejection in the last few years will likely improve short- and long-term outcomes; results from trials of new agents such as eculizumab and bortezomib, which may improve outcomes in this group, are eagerly awaited.

Surgical techniques in living donation have undergone a revolution in recent years, with minimally invasive procurement (laparoscopic approach) becoming the standard. Single-port laparoscopy and E-NOTES include some of the recent advances in this area. Robotic assistance has been used and may become more common as the next generation of robots appears, with haptic feedback and cost-efficient and less-cumbersome equipment.

Intestinal transplantation, especially in combination with liver or as part of a multivisceral transplant, is now a viable procedure with good results, and has dramatically improved the lives of many recipients, a large number of whom are children. Short-term outcomes are excellent, but in the longer term, rejection, sepsis, and post-transplant lymphoproliferative disorder (PTLD) remain problematic and ongoing efforts are needed to manage these patients. Living-donor intestinal transplantation remains in its infancy, but improvements in the diagnosis of rejection, reduction in chronic allograft damage, and the use of cell-based therapy all hold promise for the future.

Living-donor liver transplantation has become increasingly frequent over the last decade, with over 4000 such operations in the USA alone. Concerns over donor morbidity and mortality remain, and debate exists over which liver lobe to use, but this procedure has undoubtedly been life-saving for many. Short- and long-term donor outcomes that are direct indicators of donor safety will no doubt be the primary determinant of widespread application of adult-to-adult live-donor liver transplantation. The National Institutes of Health (NIH)-sponsored A2ALL study has provided and will continue to provide comprehensive data on this important issue.

Solid-organ pancreas transplantation is now considered a routine operation, with 1-year graft survival rates of 95% for simultaneous kidney–pancreas transplantation. Many centers are now extending the previously strict criteria for donors, with older, obese, or donation-after-cardiac-death (DCD) donors being increasingly used. Early evidence from single-center studies suggests good results in these cases, but careful monitoring of longer-term outcomes is essential. Living-donor pancreas transplantation—successfully pioneered at the University of Minnesota—has not become widely used in the last few years, largely due to concerns about donor morbidity, coupled with relatively short waiting times for deceased-donor pancreata. Live donors for pancreas could become important in the future if successful islet transplantation increases the demand for pancreata, thus prolonging wait times. Recipient selection has also been broadened, with some type-2 diabetics (nonobese obligatory insulin-dependent individuals) undergoing transplantation, with excellent outcomes.

A little over a decade ago, the landmark publication by the Edmonton group suggested that islet-cell transplantation, with excellent short-term results, could be a viable option for treatment of diabetes mellitus. Subsequent outcomes have shown that all the problems facing islet-cell transplantation have not yet been solved, with multiple donors required, relatively low long-term insulin-free survival, and difficulties in monitoring rejection. Progress has been hampered by the fact that donor organs used in islet transplantation are often of poorer quality than solid-organ transplants, and rejection is difficult to monitor. Currently a niche for islet-cell transplantation has been created, with those with hypoglycemic unawareness and low insulin requirements most likely to benefit from cell-based therapy. It seems probable, however, that future developments will lead to significant progress in islet transplantation, with experiments involving encapsulation, alternative implantation sites, and calcineurin-inhibitor-free regimens all underway. Attempts to use stem-cell therapy to generate islets—preferably with the recipient phenotype—continue, and this remains a fast-changing and exciting field.

Stem cells have already been used to repair damaged tissue in humans and have allowed novel transplantation techniques, such as stem-cell-derived laryngeal transplantation. In rat models, stem cells can be induced into primitive kidneys, which can be implanted into the peritoneal cavity and then produce urine. Hemapoetic stem cells have been infused into recipients using a combined bone-marrow and renal transplant, with resulting tolerance in a small number of individuals. Cell-based therapy is perhaps poised to unlock a huge potential in transplantation, with improved organ repair, organ neogenesis, and the induction of tolerance by either the generation of donor-derived cells or the creation of chimerism in the recipient.

After the rapid improvements in outcomes in the 1990s, related to the introduction of mycophenylate mofetil and tacrolimus, it may seem as if recent progress in immunosuppressive regimens has been comparatively slow. However, we believe that the early 21st century is likely to witness exciting changes, as we recognize that the immune system requires coaxing and persuasion rather than aggressive domination. New calcineurin-free regimens, such as those including alefacept and tofacitinib, are under trial, and the importance of B-cell depletion—and its effect on long-term outcomes, such as chronic antibody-mediated rejection—is increasingly being recognized. Modern techniques also allow us to target allograft endothelial cells with more precision, for example by perfusing agents which bind to these cells into the organ on the back table prior to transplantation. Furthermore, the development of ex vivo normothermic perfusion techniques may allow maintenance of the organ for a long enough period to permit manipulation of the donor endothelial cell so that the recipient's immune system does not "see" foreign HLA or other antigens.

It is difficult to predict which of these exciting and often dramatic experiments will realize the enormous hope and effort invested in them by the transplant community. It is certainly possible, perhaps likely, that readers of this book two decades from now will ridicule many of the ideas described and ask why we could not see now, what to them has since become obvious. That may be part of the fun, but this much is clear: we are highly privileged to be working in a field where change is a certainty, where the effects of that change on the lives of our patients will surely be profound, and where that change is driven by the desire to improve the lives of a great number of individuals across the world. Most of all, we are privileged to work in a field where, with an unceasing repetition that is never unappreciated, our patients and their families confer their trust upon and invest their hopes within us.

Index

Prepared by: Dr Laurence Errington

Note: Page numbers in *italics* refer to Figures; those in **bold** to Tables.

Abdominal Organ Transplantation: State of the Art, First Edition.
Edited by Nizam Mamode and Raja Kandaswamy.
© 2013 Blackwell Publishing Ltd. Published 2013 by Blackwell Publishing Ltd.